Fast Facts

Fast Facts: Depression

Third edition

WITHDRAWN

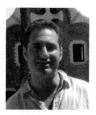

Mark Haddad PhD RGN RMN
Clinical Research Fellow
Institute of Psychiatry at King's College London
and South London and Maudsley
NHS Foundation Trust, London, UK

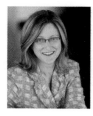

Jane Gunn PhD MBBS DRANZCOG FRACGP
Chair, Primary Care Research
Head, Department of General Practice
Melbourne Medical School
University of Melbourne, Australia

Declaration of Independence
This book is as balanced and as practical as we can make it.
Ideas for improvement are always welcome: feedback@fastfacts.com

✝ HEALTH PRESS

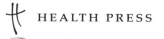

Fast Facts: Depression
First published 2003; second edition 2005
Third edition August 2011

Text © 2011 Mark Haddad, Jane Gunn
© 2011 in this edition Health Press Limited
Health Press Limited, Elizabeth House, Queen Street, Abingdon,
Oxford OX14 3LN, UK
Tel: +44 (0)1235 523233
Fax: +44 (0)1235 523238

Book orders can be placed by telephone or via the website.
For regional distributors or to order via the website, please go to:
www.fastfacts.com
For telephone orders, please call +44 (0)1752 202301 (UK, Europe and Asia–
Pacific), 1 800 247 6553 (USA, toll free) or +1 419 281 1802 (Americas).

Fast Facts is a trademark of Health Press Limited.

A CIP record for this title is available from the British Library.

ISBN 978-1-905832-86-6

Haddad M (Mark)
Fast Facts: Depression/
Mark Haddad, Jane Gunn

Typesetting and page layout by Zed, Oxford, UK.
Printed by Latimer Trend & Company Ltd, Plymouth, UK.

Text printed on biodegradable and recyclable paper
manufactured using elemental chlorine free (ECF) wood
pulp from well-managed forests.

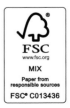

Introduction

Depression is a disorder of mood, so mysteriously painful and elusive in the way it becomes known to the self – to the mediating intellect – as to verge close to being beyond description. It thus remains nearly incomprehensible to those who have not experienced it in its extreme mode, although the gloom, 'the blues' which people go through occasionally and associate with the general hassle of everyday existence are of such prevalence that they do give many individuals a hint of the illness in its catastrophic form

William Styron, *Darkness Visible*, 1990

Depression is one of the commonest mental disorders of the 21st century, both in the developing world and in industrialized societies. An estimated 151 million people currently suffer from this disorder worldwide. Its prevalence has been examined within the general population, among primary care attendees and in people experiencing other health problems. It affects around 1 in 6 men and 1 in 4 women at some time in their lives, and in any 12-month period around 5% of people in the community are depressed.

Depression is more prevalent in women than men, and it is more common among people who have been separated from partners and people of lower socioeconomic status. Although it is one of the most widespread mental health problems in all settings that have been investigated, its distribution varies between nations, and is often higher in urban than in rural environments.

For around half of those people who experience depression, it occurs as a single episode, usually lasting between 3 and 9 months. However, for many people the condition is experienced as recurrent episodes or ongoing symptoms. Depression has a profound impact on social and economic mobility through increased disability and absenteeism from work; these effects on function and social inclusion are closely related to depression recurrence and chronicity.

People with physical health problems, especially those that are chronic, painful or disabling, are at increased risk of being depressed, and this combination of physical and mental illnesses negatively affects the course and outcome of both conditions. In primary care consultations depression is among the commonest of presenting problems. Because of this frequency of occurrence and the deleterious association with medical conditions, its recognition and effective management are important for both generalist and specialist clinicians working within medicine, nursing and associated disciplines, and in primary care, medical, surgical, intermediate care and residential settings.

Because depression is such a common and major public health problem there is a vital need for clinicians' knowledge and skills to be based on robust and up-to-date evidence and appropriate systems of service delivery. This book has been written by independent clinician researchers with the needs of busy health professionals working in these settings particularly in mind. We present to you some of the latest thinking about the nature of depression and the complex issues that surround the identification and management of the problem. We also provide you with concise and clear descriptions of the features, risks and management of depression suitable for both primary care and specialist medical settings. We hope that *Fast Facts: Depression* provides you with an efficient way to gain an overview to the latest thinking about depression. By reading this book you will be prompted to reflect upon the way in which depression enters into many of your routine consultations and how it differs from ordinary sadness. We also provide you with guidance on evidence-based assessment and management practice at individual and organizational levels.

Etymology and history

The word depression derives (via French) from the Late Latin *deprimere*, which means to press or push down; it has many different meanings that are connected by this sense of a lower or downward inclination. Its uses as a noun within the fields of geology, economics, medicine, meteorology and psychology share this meaning of a reduced function, downturn and sunken or lower level.

A distinct condition characterized by a dejected mood has been evident in writings since antiquity, with key features alluded to in the Christian Bible (e.g. Psalms 32, 38, 143; 1Kings 19, 1–5; Job 17), and a long tradition systematized in the medical writings of Hippocrates and Galen, involving theorizing about bodily fluids called humors whose imbalance was seen as responsible for disease (Figure 1.1). A tendency towards melancholy was understood to be related to an excess of the humor associated with coldness and dryness – black bile; indeed, the term melancholia is derived from the Greek word for 'black bile'. Grief and fear were regarded as characteristic features, as well as provoking influences, for melancholia, and this concept encompassed both depression and anxiety – which were not considered or classified as separate conditions until the mid-19th century. The use of the term depression as a noun to describe low mood and a 'depression of the spirits' gradually entered usage from the 18th century. The humoral theories persisted as the dominant explanation of mood (and other) disorders until the 19th century, when the use of the term 'depression' in medical works became increasingly common, and an emphasis on the features of depression and the categorization of symptoms enabled the construction of the modern disorder of depression.

The last century has been characterized by an interplay of multiple and often competing perspectives on depression – concerning the role of environmental and intrapsychic factors, the relative importance of biological and psychological mechanisms, and the relevance of collective social and economic forces in contrast to a focus on the

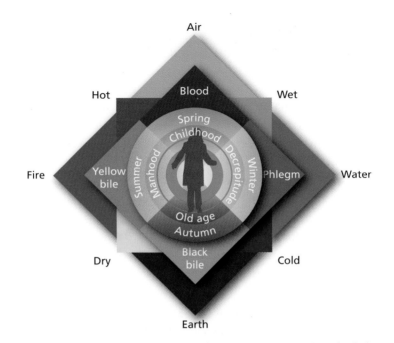

Figure 1.1 The four humors: a theory from antiquity to explain the balance between temperament, disease and the natural world.

individual. The view that depression is largely a medicalization of normal sadness has been strongly voiced in both popular and academic texts, and considerable impetus to this critique of clinical practice has been derived from massive increases in the prescribing of antidepressant drugs in the USA, UK and elsewhere over the past two decades. On the other hand, our understanding of the physiological changes and genetic markers associated with depression is rapidly advancing, with increasingly sophisticated research techniques providing a clearer picture of brain function abnormalities associated with depression and of the way that gene–environment interactions may give rise to the development of this disorder.

Debates and controversy about the meaning, origins and best ways of managing depression are by no means over; however, the past decade has seen major developments in integrating viewpoints and a particular focus on the pragmatics of clinical management and service organization.

The impact of depression

Depression has multiple impacts, affecting the subjective well-being and normal functioning of the individual and frequently interfering with the ability to work, as well as to manage social and family commitments (Table 1.1). The effects of depression are also felt by family, carers and the wider community, and the illness experience places a particular strain on relationships between partners/spouses, children and parents. There is evidence that maternal depression can have a negative effect on children – who may show deficits in social, cognitive and psychological functioning, and appear to have heightened vulnerability for depression and other mental health problems in later life.

Depression is currently ranked as the third greatest disease burden in the world, and by 2030 it is projected to be the leading cause of disability in high-income countries and the second leading cause globally. The total annual cost of depression in the member states of the European Union was estimated at €118 billion in 2004, of which around 60% was from indirect costs associated with depression morbidity and mortality. The estimated annual costs of depression in the USA are over $80 billion.

There is a strong association between depression and the increased use of health services, with depressed patients using significantly more

TABLE 1.1

The effects of depression

- Individual suffering, distress and poor life quality
- Increased risk of suicide
- Reduced well-being of families and friends
- Absenteeism and reduced work productivity
- Increased medical care costs – approximately doubled for people with depression compared with matched controls
- Negative interactions with medical problems – worsened illness course, increased disability and increased mortality
- Increased all-cause mortality

general medical services than non-depressed peers, so that the total healthcare costs are between 50% and 100% higher for those who are depressed.

Depression occurs frequently in combination with chronic physical illness, and this combination or comorbidity adversely affects the course and outcome of both disorders. Depression combined with long-term illness also causes greater disability, more extensive loss of productivity and greater increases in healthcare costs, and it is associated with more treatment complications and elevated mortality.

The risk of suicide for individuals with a history of depression is more than double that for the general population. Around 60% of people who commit suicide have had depression, and younger people who kill themselves often have an alcohol or substance misuse disorder in addition to being depressed. Although women are more likely to experience depression than men, in most of the world men are much more likely to commit suicide than women; in industrialized countries the suicide risk among men is two to four times higher than for women.

Changes in prevalence

A number of studies have identified increases in depression prevalence during the 20th century, and commentators have been prompted to talk of a 'depression epidemic' afflicting industrialized societies. However, study findings concerning increased rates of depression are equivocal – although increases have often been identified by means of comparing cross-sectional studies, these are generally not found in longitudinal studies of depression prevalence within well-defined populations. Additionally, epidemiological surveys often make use of participant recall of the experience of prior mental disorder, which may be subject to recall errors. While there is some evidence that onset is occurring at younger ages and there may be increases in depression incidence overall, it seems that the extent of any increase in prevalence has been overstated. When studies adopt concurrent assessment rather than retrospective recall and the findings of appropriate studies are pooled, there appears to be no evidence for increases in child or adolescent depression between the mid-1960s and mid-1990s. For adult depression, reviews indicate an increase in rates of depression during the period between 1960 and 1975, with mixed findings over subsequent years.

What has definitely changed is public awareness of this disorder, the number of people who seek treatment, the volume of prescriptions for antidepressant medications and the perception of healthcare professionals, as shown by the growth in the scientific literature on this topic. It is likely that a range of influences, including campaigns to improve the understanding of depression, the growth of talking treatments for psychological problems and increases in suicide rates – particularly among younger people in industrialized countries in the 1980s and 1990s – may well have added to the general awareness and concern about mood disorders.

Challenges for assessment and management

The concept of depression poses considerable challenges for clinicians and the public: the diagnosis may be legitimately used across a wide array of presentations, yet diagnosing a person with depression may not necessarily help them or their family or carers to identify the best way of approaching their problems. The diagnosis of depression has, at its heart, features of distress, sadness and dejection, which are – to some extent – part of the human condition. Although these are negative experiences that impair function, they may nonetheless be evaluated in diverse ways by individuals and their cultures. There are valid concerns that the breadth of severity encompassed by current diagnostic symptoms may lead to an overdiagnosis of depression. A low threshold for diagnosis risks normal emotional states being inappropriately treated as a medical condition, which may inhibit appropriate means of adjustment and recovery.

However, there are well-justified contrary concerns too. Despite being one of the leading causes of disability worldwide, many people need, but do not receive, treatment for depression. The stigma surrounding mental illnesses and a lack of understanding of this condition together with negative attitudes towards its treatments are important barriers to seeking treatment. There is good evidence that depression is often not recognized by clinicians, and that even when it's identified it is frequently inadequately managed by health services in the USA, UK and other countries. Research indicates that 30–50% of depression cases are missed in primary care and it appears that recognition problems are amplified by the presence of comorbid medical conditions, which complicate the help-seeking and assessment processes.

Knowledge about depression and its management has developed significantly since the latter half of the 20th century. A range of treatments are available, with a robust evidence base indicating that both psychopharmacological and psychosocial approaches are likely to be beneficial, together with growing evidence for particular models of service organization and delivery involving methods for case identification, for linking between primary and specialist mental health service providers, and for coordinating individualized care across healthcare sectors. Alongside professionally delivered treatments, there have been important developments in self-help and guided self-help approaches that may make use of a range of media such as books, the internet, telephones and audio materials. Despite very significant progress, there remain obstacles to treatment delivery – in many settings there are shortages of professionals trained in the delivery of evidence-based psychological treatments, and in many countries effective depression management is impeded by problems in the structures or funding arrangements of health services. Additionally, although there has been considerable growth in our knowledge of the causes, course and management of depression, there remain gaps in our understanding. Although the overwhelming majority of patients with depression are managed within primary care, much of the evidence and resulting clinical guidance is derived from studies in secondary and tertiary sectors.

At a fundamental level there remain important questions and uncertainties about the best way to understand and classify depression. A central debate about the relative merits of categorical (case or non-case based on a specific pattern of symptoms) or dimensional (based on measures of symptom severity or prior illness course) approaches to classification is particularly relevant to this disorder. A continuity between milder forms of depression and fully symptomatic disorder appears in community studies that have examined course and correlates for a range of presentations. Depression that does not meet the full criteria for a formal diagnosis is increasingly recognized to cause considerable suffering and places a significant burden on the healthcare system; it is also related to increased mortality and is a risk factor for future major depression. Developing useful approaches to understand and assist people who experience depressive symptoms across the spectrum of presentations remains a central goal. Consensus and clinical evidence is strongest for the more severe forms of depression, but important questions remain about the best ways of understanding and helping the many people who are affected by milder mood problems and of how to provide efficient and robustly evidence-based support that does not simplistically medicalize life's problems.

Key points – overview

- Depression has been evident as a problem for individuals and societies since antiquity – but public and professional awareness has markedly increased over the past quarter of a century.
- Although much progress has been made in clarifying the clinical features and distribution of depression within populations, significant debate remains and there are ongoing difficulties about how to best understand and manage depression, particularly in its milder forms.
- Improved knowledge about the features, course and management of depression has enabled more prompt recognition, evidence-based treatment decisions and improved outcomes.

Key references

Blazer DG. Depression in late life: review and commentary. *J Gerontol A Biol Sci Med Sci* 2003;58:249–65.

Dowrick C. *Beyond Depression: A New Approach to Understanding and Management*, 2nd edn. Oxford: OUP, 2009.

World Health Organization. *The World Health Report 2001 – Mental Health: New Understanding, New Hope*. Geneva: WHO, 2001. Available from www.who.int/whr/2001/en, last accessed 15 July 2011.

World Health Organization. *The Global Burden of Disease: 2004 Update*. Geneva: WHO, 2008. Available from www.who.int/healthinfo/global_burden_disease/2004_report_update/en/index.html, last accessed 15 July 2011.

A quiet mind cureth all them, but all they cannot comfort a distressed soul: who can put to silence the voice of desperation? All that is single in other melancholy, Horribile, dirum, pestilens, atrox, ferum, concur in this, it is more than melancholy in the highest degree; a burning fever of the soul; so mad, saith Jacchinus, by this misery; fear, sorrow, and despair, he puts for ordinary symptoms of melancholy. They are in great pain and horror of mind, distraction of soul, restless, full of continual fears, cares, torments, anxieties, they can neither eat, drink, nor sleep for them, take no rest

Robert Burton, *The Anatomy of Melancholy*, 1621

Problems defining depression

'Depression', within medicine and the health sciences, refers to a spectrum of mood disturbances that range from mild to severe and from short-lived episodes to unremitting illness. Diagnosis is based on the symptom picture as well as the severity, duration and course of the disease. It is characterized by low mood and the absence of positive affect (loss of interest and enjoyment in ordinary activities), together with a range of associated emotional, cognitive, physical and behavioral features. However, depression is a heterogeneous condition and although classification systems have usefully clarified the process of clinical diagnosis, uncertainties remain about the validity of accepted diagnostic thresholds and even about the best means of conceptualizing depression.

The validity of the concept of depression is questioned on a range of counts. Much of the debate hinges on the basis for defining depression as a disease entity and the associated difficulty identifying a natural boundary between this construct and normality or the range of accepted responses to the various forms of human loss. Depression, like most psychiatric disorders, is defined by its syndrome or symptom

15

profile. In this respect, psychiatry is in the position occupied by most of medicine 200 years ago of delineating conditions by their symptoms and lacking clear evidence of distinct causal or fundamental defining characteristics based on specific pathological, physiological or chromosomal abnormality.

Alongside the lack of clear causal and confirmatory biological characteristics for depression (as well as for a large number of other psychiatric conditions), there is a problem of where to draw the boundary, as the characteristic features are continuously distributed within the population. The distinction between depression and the distress and angst that are a part of normal human experience requires a dichotomization of this continuum of symptoms. Rather than being based on 'hard' criteria related to a clear causal mechanism, with associated biological markers, this differentiation is made on the basis of clinical, prognostic and operational considerations. Although this is problematic, it is useful to bear in mind that this applies to such commonly occurring medical conditions as diabetes, hypertension and irritable bowel syndrome, where the variation between extensive and disabling symptoms and few and insignificant symptoms appears to be continuous.

As well as problems defining the boundaries of depression, there are difficulties delineating it from other mental disorders. In the community, as well as in primary care settings, the most prevalent mood disorder is a combination of depression and anxiety. The overlap between symptoms such as low mood, lack of energy, insomnia, worry and irritability is considerable, with nearly 9% of the UK household population, for example, suffering from this subthreshold combination to a clinically significant extent. Among people who meet the diagnostic thresholds for depression or anxiety disorders there is also a high degree of co-occurrence of these conditions, raising questions about the specificity of these diagnostic categories.

There is no distinct etiology for depression. A common genetic factor for anxiety and depressive conditions is apparent, and similarities in the types of environmental adversities that seem to provoke depression and anxiety, such as physical or sexual abuse and neglect in childhood, have been reported. Moreover, the pharmacological treatments principally classified as antidepressants are also effective in anxiety disorders, and similar types of individual, group and computer-assisted psychological treatments appear effective for both conditions.

Some investigators and commentators have questioned the validity of depression on the basis of supposed cultural variations that exist in its presentation, prevalence, prognosis and meaning within different cultures. Some commentators identify psychiatric diagnoses such as depression as 'Western' categories that can be imposed on non-Western peoples – a form of medical imperialism.

There are then fundamental problems in the notion of depression as a psychiatric disorder. But where does this leave us? There are some important aspects of validity adopted from psychometric theory that are relevant to considering the robustness of the concept of depression as a disorder: there is good evidence of the concurrent and predictive validity of this diagnosis; the diagnosis is associated consistently with disability, reduced quality of life and particular service needs; and there is likewise an extensive literature indicating the suffering that is associated with the condition and the natural history of the illness, its response to various treatments and its relationship to other conditions.

Despite some very real questions about the central validity of the concept of depression, there is little doubt among researchers and clinicians that this classification (like most psychiatric diagnoses) is very useful, if not invaluable. The diagnostic entity of depression allows clear communication between researchers, clinicians, service developers and providers as well as services users and carers; it also enables us to develop greater understanding through international research that will provide richer and more precise detail of etiology and risk, illness course, and management and treatment. It is inconceivable that these activities could persist in the absence of clear criteria for this condition based upon the presence of particular symptoms. A consensus currently exists that the many benefits of applying the classification system for depression, as for other psychiatric conditions, outweigh the disadvantages.

Diagnosis

The cluster of symptoms experienced in depression is central to its classification as a mental disorder. The number, intensity and effects of these symptoms are central to differentiating depression from normal experiences and from other disorders. There is a consensus concerning the symptoms of depression. The two most widely used diagnostic systems are the World Health Organization (WHO) International Classification of Diseases and Related Health Problems, currently in its tenth revision (ICD-10), and the Diagnostic and Statistical Manual of Mental Disorders of the American Psychiatric Association, currently in its fourth edition (DSM-IV). The criteria used by these classification systems are broadly similar, though the symptom thresholds differ; it is likely that the small number of differences that exist will be reduced in further revisions. The DSM-IV criteria will be used as the basis for clinical descriptions of depression and the related disorders considered in this book. This is because the majority of research and the most recent clinical guidelines that inform knowledge about depression and its management use the DSM criteria.

Major depressive disorder

The central condition of 'depression' is 'major depressive disorder' in the DSM-IV classification, and is experienced as a single or recurrent episode. Within ICD-10, it is simply called 'depressive episode' or 'recurrent depressive episode'. The terms 'clinical depression' and 'unipolar depression' are often also used.

A diagnosis of (major) depression is based on a person experiencing a particular group of unpleasant symptoms affecting mood, thinking, motivation and physical functions that are persistent and have clear effects on the person's ability to conduct their normal activities. As shown in Table 2.1, the cardinal features of low mood and diminished interest are central to the condition, and at least one of these has to be present for a diagnosis to be made. In addition to these core symptoms, a minimum number of additional depressive symptoms are required, such that at least five of the group of nine symptoms are present in total (Table 2.1). Symptoms should:

- have been present for at least 2 weeks, during which time they have

TABLE 2.1

The symptoms of major depressive disorder, single episode

- A total of at least **five out of nine** symptoms must be present
- Symptoms are pervasive, sustained and impair the person's usual function
- Symptoms are experienced for most of the day, for most days for at least 2 weeks
- One or both of these symptoms must be present:
  1) low mood
  2) markedly diminished interest and pleasure ('anhedonia')
- In addition, further symptoms, also experienced nearly every day, are necessary for a diagnosis:
  3) reduced energy or fatigue (anergia)
  4) disturbed sleep (insomnia or hypersomnia)
  5) agitation or slowed down speech or movement (psychomotor agitation or retardation)
  6) disturbed appetite (may be increased or decreased, and may be accompanied by significant weight loss)
  7) feelings of guilt or worthlessness
  8) reduced concentration
  9) recurrent thoughts of death or suicidal ideas

been experienced for much of the day for every day or nearly every day
- represent a change from the person's usual presentation, causing significant distress and negatively impacting on functioning.

As a syndrome of this sort may occur during normal bereavement, or may be triggered by the effects of a health condition or of prescribed or illicit medication, these situations are specified as exclusionary criteria, and if present should prevent the diagnosis of depression being reached.

Single episode or recurrent. A generation ago, standard psychiatry texts typically considered depression as an acute illness best managed by specialist treatment. The findings of longitudinal naturalistic studies have increasingly revealed the variability of illness course and show that, for many people, depression has a lifelong episodic course, characterized by relapses. There is consistent evidence from population-based studies (as well as primary- and specialist-care samples) that around 50% of people who have an initial depressive episode will have further episodes. Each episode of depression increases the risks for additional episodes, with a 70% risk of relapse following two episodes and a 90% risk after three. People with a history of depression have been found to have, on average, between five and nine further episodes during their lifetime.

Chronic depression. Depression is experienced as a chronic unremitting disorder by 10–20% of people. Diagnostic criteria define chronic depression as a minimum 2-year history of meeting the symptom threshold for a major depressive episode.

Severity. As well as specifying whether depressive disorder is a single episode, recurrent or chronic, the severity of the current episode is an important clinical descriptor. Severity is clarified from the number and intensity of symptoms, with categorization as shown in Table 2.2.

There are further specifiers for depressive disorder that concern the pattern and intensity of the symptoms experienced; the most relevant are outlined here.

TABLE 2.2

Classification of severity of depressive disorder

- **Mild depression:** few, if any, symptoms above the five necessary for diagnosis,* with these symptoms resulting in only minor impairment of function
- **Moderate depression:** the symptoms and functional impairment experienced are between the 'mild' and 'severe' categorizations
- **Severe depression:** involves most of the symptoms,* and these markedly interfere with the person's functioning

*See Table 2.1.

Psychotic features. The experience of abnormal perceptions (hallucinations) or beliefs (delusions) may be part of the presentation in a severe episode of depressive disorder. This is part of the symptom picture for around 15% of people who fulfill the criteria for a major depressive episode, providing a 0.4% lifetime risk for major depression with psychotic features. These features are particularly associated with experiencing feelings of worthlessness or guilt and may often share the themes of self-deprecation and blame; they are a serious aspect of presentation and may interfere with the individual's ability to make sound judgments in a way that puts them at increased risk of harming themselves. The presence of psychotic symptoms is a strong indication that specialist multiprofessional management is required, possibly including inpatient assessment and treatment.

Melancholic features. 'Melancholia' remains an important aspect of the features and presentation of depression. It refers to a generally severe presentation in which there is pervasive anhedonia – the loss of interest or pleasure is extreme, with a complete or near-complete lack of reactivity of mood to positive events. There is a pattern of the depressed mood that is substantially worse in the morning (diurnal variation). Sleep is disturbed, with the person waking early in the morning and being unable to get back to sleep. Psychomotor retardation or agitation is likely to be pronounced, and significant appetite and weight loss and excessive or inappropriate guilt are characteristic of this subtype.

Seasonal affective disorder (SAD) occurs when depression recurrences follow a seasonal pattern. Rather than a separate diagnosis, this is a specific category of major depression (and so the person must meet depression diagnosis criteria). DSM-IV criteria for this particular pattern of recurrent major depressive disorder specify that:
- depressive episodes occur repeatedly at a particular time of the year
- remissions between episodes occur at a particular time of the year
- two major depressive episodes must have occurred exhibiting this seasonal pattern during the past 2 years, with no non-seasonal episodes in this period

- seasonal depressive episodes outnumber other depressive episodes
during the individual's lifetime.

Typically, episodes occur during the winter months and are characterized by decreased activity and reduced energy, and withdrawal from social activity, together with atypical depressive symptoms – most usually increased sleep and cravings for carbohydrates, leading to weight gain. Although the geographic distribution of SAD has not been rigorously studied, evidence suggests that SAD is more prevalent in Northern latitudes. The validity of SAD is less well accepted in Europe than in the USA, and the ICD-10 has only provisional criteria for research.

Postpartum depression is not a separate mood disorder from major depression. The term specifies important diagnostic information about onset of the depressive episode, which diagnostic criteria specify must be within 4 weeks of giving birth to a child. Around 10–15% of new mothers may be affected.

Many women experience the 'baby blues', emotional disturbances following childbirth characterized by tearfulness, mood swings, irritability and sleep disturbances, which characteristically arise in the first week after delivery. These are mild and transient mood disturbances that may affect more than half of all mothers and resolve spontaneously. A diagnosis of depressive disorder with postpartum onset requires the presence and duration of the depression symptoms and consequent impairment described for major depressive disorder.

Dysthymic disorder

Dysthymic disorder is a form of depression characterized by both its persistence – it is a chronic illness, with features persisting for at least 2 years – and by the symptom picture, which involves fewer and less serious symptoms than major depression (Table 2.3).

In contrast to depression, the symptoms of dysthymia do not necessarily cause significant functional impairment within social, occupational or other domains. Dysthymia is associated with an increased risk of subsequent major depression, and may be a cause of considerable social disability or of unhealthy lifestyle choices.

TABLE 2.3

Symptoms of dysthymic disorder

For diagnostic purposes at least two of these symptoms must be experienced for most of the day, for more days than not, for at least 2 years

- Disturbed sleep – insomnia or hypersomnia
- Poor concentration or difficulty making decisions
- Reduced energy or fatigue (anergia)
- Disturbed appetite – may be increased or decreased
- Feelings of hopelessness or pessimism
- Low self-esteem

In the USA the term 'double depression' is sometimes used to describe the occurrence of major depressive episodes supervening upon a background of dysthymia.

Subthreshold or subclinical depression

Additionally, the category of subthreshold (or subclinical) depression – called 'minor depression' in the DSM-IV (where it is noted as a potential rather than formal diagnosis that requires further empirical validation) – is used when an individual has two to four depressive symptoms, including depressed mood or loss of interest or pleasure, during a 2-week period but has not had these symptoms for 2 years (as this would otherwise meet the criteria for dysthymia). This categorization also excludes individuals with a previous history of major depressive disorder. Studies of episode duration and frequency, family history and associated impairments indicate that subthreshold depression is part of a continuum of depression severity, and that it is associated with a greater risk of developing major depressive disorder. Role impairments, distress and risk of progression to a major depressive episode are clear reasons to support the serious consideration of subthreshold presentations of depression, but at the same time concerns about medicalizing distress are particularly relevant to the use of a specific diagnostic category for this level of problematic symptoms.

Mixed anxiety and depressive disorder

Depression and anxiety disorders frequently coexist, with community studies consistently identifying a substantial proportion of people either currently meeting the diagnostic criteria for, or having a lifetime history of, both conditions. The strong association between lifetime risks for anxiety disorders and major depression means that if an individual has one of these disorders, they have a 25–50% chance of developing the other disorder.

As well as coexisting conditions that meet respective diagnostic criteria, there appears to be a substantial prevalence of depression and anxiety conditions which, though clinically significant, do not have associated symptoms to an extent that justifies a diagnosis if considered separately. This combination of depression and anxiety symptoms of limited and equal intensity is termed 'mixed anxiety and depressive disorder' (Table 2.4). Although it is noted in both classification systems, it remains a subsyndromal diagnosis in the

TABLE 2.4

Features of mixed anxiety and depressive disorder

- Diagnosis based on the presence of symptoms of anxiety and depression, but neither is clearly predominant
- Neither type of symptom is present to the extent that justifies a diagnosis if considered separately
- Symptoms should be present for at least 4 weeks, and result in significant distress or functional impairment
- Typical symptoms include those listed below

Anxiety	Depression
Persistent nervousness	Sleep disturbance
Palpitations, chest pain, dizziness	Fatigue or low energy
Irritability	Hopelessness or pessimism
Fearful anticipation	Poor concentration
Excessive alertness	Low self-esteem or feelings of worthlessness

ICD-10 (where it is considered among other anxiety disorders) and a provisional diagnosis in DSM-IV (diagnostic criteria are noted in an appendix rather than the main text). International studies have provided conflicting evidence in relation to the prevalence and stability of this condition, and research is hampered by uncertainties about diagnostic criteria, with the ICD-10 offering vague guidance and the DSM-IV considered overly restrictive by some commentators.

There are considerable uncertainties about this categorization – although on the one hand it may help to identify and develop improved ways of assisting people with common and distressing mental health problems, it appears to extend the boundaries of our notions of mental disorder, and hence involves a medicalization of human distress.

Adjustment disorder

Depression is differentiated from adjustment disorder, which is a rather broad and ill-defined category comprising the emotional or behavioral response to a stressful event, characterized by marked distress or clearly reduced social functioning. Although features vary, they include one or a combination of depressed mood, anxiety or worry. The effects do not persist beyond a 6-month period, and the precipitating stressful event does not include bereavement.

Bipolar disorder

An important distinction is made between unipolar forms of depression such as major depression and dysthymia which involve persistent low moods, and bipolar depression, in which the mood alternates between emotional extremes or poles, with bouts of low moods followed by extreme highs or mania. 'Manic depression', a term first used in the late 19th century, was initially applied to this condition. While unipolar forms of depression are more common in women than in men, bipolar disorder affects men and women equally, and is far less common than depressive disorder, affecting about 5 people in 1000, with a lifetime risk of around 1% (although around 5% may experience subthreshold symptoms or bipolar spectrum disorder).

Diagnosis is based on the person experiencing an episode of abnormally and persistently elevated or irritable mood (Table 2.5). Key features of this mood disturbance center upon inflated self-esteem or grandiose ideas, a decreased need for sleep and increased mental and physical activity, involving over-talkativeness and racing thoughts. The person's attention span is often reduced and there is a tendency to engage in reckless and uncharacteristic behavior – such as spending sprees, extravagant or impractical schemes, sexual indiscretions, gambling or substance misuse. Behavior may become intolerant or aggressive, and in extreme forms of a manic state the person may experience psychotic features – delusions and hallucinations – that are usually congruent with the person's disturbed mood. The commonest psychotic symptom in bipolar disorder is grandiose delusions, but paranoid delusions or exaggerated mistrust and suspicion of others are often present; other psychotic symptoms may occur, including thought disorder, hallucinations and mood-incongruent psychotic symptoms.

TABLE 2.5

Diagnostic features of bipolar disorder

- A distinct period of abnormally and persistently elevated or irritable mood, lasting at least 1 week (or 4 days for hypomania/bipolar II disorder)
- The mood change is severe enough to disrupt normal activities
- Several of the following symptoms are present:
  - inflated self-esteem or grandiosity
  - decreased requirements for sleep
  - racing thoughts or flight of ideas
  - reduced attention or distractibility
  - increased talkativeness
  - increased activity levels or agitation
  - increased involvement in activities that have a risk of adverse consequences (sexual relationships, business ventures, spending sprees)

In the ICD-10 classification, bipolar affective disorder is diagnosed on the basis of more than a single episode of elevated mood, which is categorized as mania or the less extreme form, hypomania. Depressive episodes are a very common part of this condition, but are not regarded as essential for diagnosis within this classification.

In the DSM-IV classification system, there are two disorder types: bipolar I disorder and bipolar II disorder. Bipolar I disorder involves the occurrence of one or more manic episodes or mixed episodes – involving a combination of the features of mania and depressive disorder – nearly every day, lasting for at least 1 week. Although individuals will often also have had one or more major depressive episodes, these are not necessary for a diagnosis.

In bipolar II disorder, the person experiences an episode of hypomania rather than mania. Additionally, at least one major depressive episode must have been experienced.

Although the diagnostic criteria specify a short minimum duration of elevated mood, this usually lasts for between 2 weeks and 5 months, with a median duration of around 4 months.

See also *Fast Facts: Bipolar Disorder.*

Key points – definitions and diagnosis

- The diagnosis of depression is problematic – primarily in relation to the validity of distinguishing this state from normal human responses to loss and trauma.
- Depression occurs at a range of severities and may often be experienced in combination with other mental disorders such as anxiety; this can be an additional source of difficulty in diagnosis.
- Widely used diagnostic criteria enable agreement about the types of symptoms and the level of severity and persistence that comprise depressive disorder.
- The diagnosis of depression involves the presence of at least one core symptom together with other associated symptoms that are experienced most of the day, for most days, for a period of at least 2 weeks.
- Depression severity is an important part of its clinical description (informing treatment decisions), and is based on the number of symptoms and their severity and effect on function.
- Depression may involve single or recurrent episodes or it may be chronic; it may also be characterized by particular features (psychotic, melancholic) or patterns of onset (seasonal, postnatal).

Key references

American Psychiatric Association. *Diagnostic and Statistical Manual of Mental Disorders, 4th edn: DSM-IV.* Arlington: American Psychiatric Publishing, 1994.

Gavin NI, Gaynes BN, Lohr KN et al. Perinatal depression: a systematic review of prevalence and incidence. *Obstet Gynecol* 2005;106:1071–83.

Goodwin G, Sachs G. *Fast Facts: Bipolar Disorder, 2nd edn.* Oxford: Health Press, 2010.

World Health Organization. *The ICD-10 for Classification of Mental and Behavioural Disorders: Clinical Descriptions and Diagnostic Guidelines.* Geneva: WHO, 1992.

I am now the most miserable man living. If what I feel were equally distributed to the whole human family, there would not be one cheerful face on the earth. Whether I shall ever be better I cannot tell; I awfully forebode I shall not. To remain as I am is impossible; I must die or be better, it appears to me

Abraham Lincoln, from personal
correspondence to family lawyer, 1842

The onset of depression, like that of many non-communicable conditions, is related to a combination of genetic, behavioral and socioeconomic environmental factors. Such risk factors for depression include: a family history of depression (genetic); alcohol misuse and violence or abuse (behavioral); and poverty (socioeconomic). Some of the risk factors for development may be modifiable (for instance, social support, employment, abuse, relationships, substance misuse), while others are not (sex, ethnic group and age, for example) and these can affect vulnerability to depression in the light of potentially precipitating events (such as negative life events).

Risk factors place an individual at a greater likelihood of developing depression, but do not predict onset with any certainty. Importantly, they provide the potential for prevention and early intervention by public health and personal health measures – which may change disorder patterns for individuals and populations.

Prevalence

Major depression. The prevalence of depression is reported differently in some studies, and some of the areas of difference are summarized in Table 3.1.

Lifetime prevalence and risk in adults. The most recent nationally representative survey of mental disorders in the USA (the National

TABLE 3.1

Differences in methods used in studies of depression prevalence

The time period over which the disorder is recorded: for instance, point prevalence, period prevalence (such as 12-month prevalence and lifetime prevalence) or risk are all commonly reported, and clearly will provide differing values within the same population.

The population sampled: depression prevalence varies according to age, sex, coexisting health problems, sociodemographic factors and geographic and cultural settings.

The type of disorder investigated: some studies have focused on common mental disorders as a category (including anxiety disorders, depressive disorder and mixed depression and anxiety) or on all depressive disorders (including minor depression, dysthymia and mixed depression and anxiety).

The depression measurement used: although most contemporary epidemiological studies use structured diagnostic interviews that provide both ICD-10 and DSM-IV diagnoses,* some large prevalence studies use instruments (e.g. symptom rating scales) which, though validated, may be subject to some level of measurement error.

*See page 18.

Comorbidity Survey Replication [NCS-R]) identified a lifetime prevalence of 16.6% for major depression among people aged 18 years and older, and a projected lifetime risk of 23.3% (projected with a standardized risk calculation as survey respondents may not have experienced depression but are within the risk period for first onset). The sample size (in excess of 9000 people) and study methods used provide good grounds for reliance on these estimates. These findings are generally consistent with the lifetime prevalence and risk rates identified in WHO World Mental Health (WMH) Surveys conducted over the past decade in 17 countries, although these indicate variations in rates between world regions and nations.

Twelve-month prevalence relates to whether the individual survey participant has experienced features meeting diagnostic criteria for an episode of depression at any time over the past 12-month period. The NCS-R identified a 12-month prevalence of 6.6% among adults surveyed, whilst a systematic review of depression prevalence studies has obtained a pooled 12-month prevalence of 4.1%. Similarly, a national prevalence study in Australia using comparable methods found a 1-year depression prevalence of 5.1%.

Lower estimates of age-standardized prevalence rates were provided by the WHO Global Burden of Disease (GBD) study, which involved a review of 56 studies from all six WHO regions, and estimated that 1.6% of men and 2.6% of women will experience a depressive episode in a 12-month period.

Point prevalence. A number of the surveys that examine point prevalence of depression make use of symptom-rating scales, which may be a factor in the variation in estimates found in the studies that report this rate. Studies that have used diagnostic interview methods have generally found point prevalence rates for depression in adults in the region of 2–4%. The rate obtained by structured interview (Clinical Interview Schedule–Revised [CIS-R], which covers non-psychotic symptoms experienced in the past week) in the latest (2007) household survey of psychiatric morbidity in England for depression was 2.3%.

Surveys also commonly measure 1-month prevalence rates and sometimes 2- or 1-week prevalence rates, and these will identify values broadly similar to point prevalence estimates.

Rates in older and younger people. Studies in Western countries indicate that although older people are more likely to have physical disorders with associated disability, and are more likely to face the loss of partners, friends and family, this age group suffers less from depression than younger people. The latest population study in England shows this: the prevalence of depression and other mood and anxiety disorders was found to be highest among those aged 45–54 years, but lowest in those aged 75 or older. Although depression that meets the threshold for diagnosis is less common among older people than in the younger adult population, it appears that depressive symptoms are relatively commonly experienced by older people and increase in those over the age of 80. A comprehensive review of studies has yielded a point prevalence rate of major depression in older people of 1.8%. But, when all depressive syndromes deemed clinically relevant are considered, the prevalence of depressive syndromes appears in the order of 12%.

The study of depression in children and young people has been hampered by misconceptions that depression is very rare among the young (hence it was scarcely recognized before the 1970s), and that depressed mood is a normal self-limiting part of adolescence: neither of these notions is correct. A recent nationwide epidemiological survey found that around 1% of 5–16 year-olds in England met diagnostic criteria for depression (0.2% in 5–10 year-olds and 1.4% in 11–16 year-olds), while a well-conducted systematic review of studies indicated a higher prevalence of depression among children and adolescents, 2.8% for those under 13 years and 5.6% among 13–18 year-olds.

Distribution by sex, sociodemographics and ethnicity. Depression (and anxiety disorders) occurs 1.5–2 times more commonly in adult women than in men, with the excess of depression being greater during women's reproductive years and less apparent in later life. This sex difference in prevalence is not explained in terms of differential effects of marital status, childcare or employment status.

A lower level of mental health problems experienced by married people is one of the most consistent epidemiological findings. Good evidence for this comes from a recent analysis of the WMH Surveys, (using data from cross-sectional household surveys in 15 countries, involving nearly 35 000 participants). A generally protective pattern for the mental disorders examined (depression and other mood, anxiety and substance misuse disorders) is associated with first marriage compared with being never married, but for depression this protective pattern is restricted to men, with no risk difference evident for women. It is frequently asserted that marriage is more beneficial for the mental health of men than women; although this does not appear true for many mental disorders, it is apparently correct for depression onset.

Being previously married, relative to being stably married, is strongly associated with an increased risk of onset of depression (and other mental disorders) for both sexes, though this increased risk of onset is significantly more pronounced among men.

Studies in a range of settings have identified a strong association between current or past abuse and depression. This is evident for physical violence, and for emotional and sexual abuse. In childhood, these are predictors of later depression onset, while in adulthood it is uncertain whether these adversities relate to new onset, or are linked to the recurrence and persistence of an established disorder.

Depression, like practically all health states and indicators, exhibits an inverse and continuous relation with socioeconomic position. Cross-national comparisons of data from the Americas and Europe indicate that poverty, unemployment and low educational attainment are associated with a near doubling of risk for common mental disorders when the lowest and the highest socioeconomic categories are compared. Socioeconomic adversity appears to predict the persistence of depression, with community epidemiological studies and examinations of depression management in primary care identifying this risk association. A systematic review and meta-analysis incorporating 60 prevalence, incidence and persistence studies revealed compelling evidence for the relation between socioeconomic inequality and depression, though constituent variables such as education, occupation, employment or income exerted differing influences. Moreover, although the evidence indicates that low socioeconomic status plays a causal role in depression development and persistence, there is also evidence that the association operates via depression leading to social and economic adversity.

There are inconsistent findings concerning the relationship between ethnicity and depression prevalence and incidence. In the UK and USA, psychiatric morbidity survey results are inconsistent, and confounding factors such as age structure and socioeconomic status influence findings. The most recent UK surveys found higher rates of depression and anxiety disorders in South Asian women, and the greatest sex differential in common mental disorder prevalence was within this ethnic group, with a threefold increased risk in women. Population studies carried out in the USA have generally found that non-Hispanic white people have an elevated prevalence of depression compared with African-American and Hispanic people, after controlling for the array of confounding and potentially interacting factors that are linked to ethnic grouping such as unemployment, income and social class, lone parent status, health insurance coverage, carer roles, chronic disease and disability, and perceived and actual social support. After such adjustments, Native Americans appear to have the highest rates of depression within the US population, and black and Asian people and Pacific Islanders the lowest rates. Studies of minority populations in New Zealand and Australia have found higher rates of depression in Maoris and Aboriginal peoples.

Migration is a process that, whether it occurs for political, economic, social or other reasons, is accompanied by stresses and the possibility of alienation. Several studies have identified higher rates of depression among migrants – for instance, among foreign students compared with those from the same country as the educational institution. Overall, the findings relating to different settings and populations are conflicting, relating no doubt to the complex array of factors involved that may influence the mental health of migrant peoples. There is some evidence of prevalence being limited by acculturation, with migrants fluent in the host nation language less likely to have elevated rates of depression. However, there is also evidence that disorder rates can remain high among those who migrated at an early age or were born to parents who migrated. Asylum seekers and refugees are particularly at risk of depression because of the combination of trauma and absence of social and cultural support networks that act as a buffer against the effects of these adverse experiences.

Related diagnoses

Minor or subthreshold depression. Milder forms of depression are distinguished from major depressive disorder using such terms as subsyndromal depression, subthreshold depression and minor depression. The lifetime prevalence of minor depression is approximately 7.5%. Point prevalence and 12-month prevalence rates are consistently lower than for major depression: a recent German national survey identified a 12-month prevalence of 1.8% (though when diagnostic interviewing was based solely on symptom count without clinical significance criteria, the 12-month rate was 6.8%).

Minor depression is relatively common in primary care settings and has been found to be associated with significant functional impairment and an adverse effect on the course of medical conditions. Experiencing subthreshold symptoms of depression also increases the risk of developing depression that meets full diagnostic criteria, though cohort studies have indicated that the risk of progression to major depression is highest among people who have dysthymia.

Dysthymia occurs less commonly than depression, with a typical lifetime prevalence of 6%, and a point prevalence of 1–3% obtained from surveys in the USA and European countries.

Bipolar affective disorder is far less common than depression. International population studies including the NCS-R have found broadly consistent rates for this disorder. Lifetime (and 12-month) prevalence rates are in the order of 1.0% (0.6%) for bipolar I disorder and 1.1% (0.8%) for bipolar II disorder. Subthreshold bipolar has a prevalence of 2.4% (1.4%). A recent re-evaluation of measurement of this disorder in the NCS-R has indicated that a lifetime prevalence of bipolar spectrum disorder (comprising bipolar I or II or subthreshold) is around 4%.

The median age of onset for bipolar disorder is 25 years (although the illness can start in early childhood or as late as the 40s and 50s. An equal number of men and women develop bipolar illness, and its prevalence is not related to ethnicity or social class.

Depression and anxiety. Symptoms of depression and anxiety often coexist. A high level of co-occurrence of these disorders has been consistently identified in epidemiological studies in many countries, with combined mood and anxiety conditions often more prevalent than 'pure' mood disorder in community samples of working age and older people.

In the NCS-R, people who had met lifetime criteria for major depression were more likely to also meet the lifetime criteria for an anxiety disorder than any other mental disorder – 59.2% showed this type of comorbidity. A similar proportion of people meeting criteria for 12-month depressive disorder also met criteria for 12-month anxiety disorder (57.5%).

Phobic disorders appear to be the commonest co-occurring conditions (coexisting lifetime prevalence: simple phobia, 26%; agoraphobia, 20%; social phobia, 14%; panic disorder, 13%; and obsessive–compulsive disorder, 14%). Anxiety problems most commonly arise in early life, and this remains the case when they accompany depression: the average age of onset of any lifetime anxiety disorder is 16 years and for social phobia it is 12 years among those with major depression.

The comorbidity of major depressive and anxiety disorders is associated with barriers to treatment and worse psychiatric outcomes, including treatment resistance, increased risk for suicide, greater chance for recurrence and greater use of medical resources.

Mixed anxiety and depression. This condition involves a combination of subthreshold features of both disorders, rather than the co-occurrence of both disorders at caseness level. There are inconsistencies in research findings on the prevalence of this combined disorder, with national psychiatric morbidity surveys conducted in England and other UK countries identifying this combined condition as the commonest disorder, with a prevalence of around 9% – more than double that of generalized anxiety or depression. Studies in other European countries and the USA have identified much lower rates of this combined condition, typically 1–2%. This is likely to be due to differences between the WHO's International Classification of Diseases and Related Health Problems, tenth revision (ICD-10) and the Diagnostic and Statistical Manual of Mental Disorders of the American Psychiatric Association, currently in its fourth edition (DSM-IV), as the latter system excludes this condition if the person has ever met criteria for a depressive or anxiety disorder, while many people included in this category in UK surveys will have been in partial remission from mood or anxiety disorders.

It has been found that the impact of mixed anxiety and depressive disorder on health-related quality of life is similar to that of pure anxiety and depression, and a fifth of all days off work in Britain occur in people with this disorder.

Age of onset of depression

The age of onset is an important aspect of the description and understanding of lifetime disorders. However, there are potential problems with the accuracy of findings derived from the retrospective recall required within such epidemiological surveys. The commencement of disorders with a vivid onset, such as panic disorder, appears to be recalled more reliably than those with a more gradual development like depression. Research also shows that recall concerning the *first* occurrence of an episodic condition such as depression is likely to be particularly poor.

Revised methods, test–retest qualification and reviews of the consistency of findings indicate that the results of the NCS-R are a major improvement on previous studies, though there remains a risk of bias in these estimates. The NCS-R study findings indicate the common age of onset for depression ranges between 19 and 44 years (interquartile range), with a median age of onset of 32 years (Figure 3.1). These findings are very similar to those from the

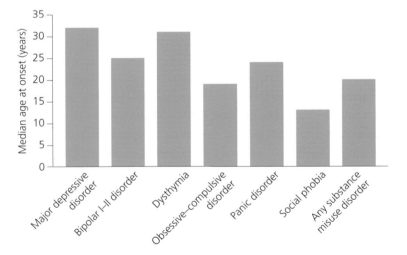

Figure 3.1 Median age of onset for common mental disorders from National Comorbidity Survey Replication data. (Based on data from Kessler RC, Berglund P, Demler O et al. Lifetime prevalence and age-of-onset distributions of DSM-IV disorders in the National Comorbidity Survey Replication. *Arch Gen Psychiatry* 2005;62:593–602.)

WHO WMH Surveys, conducted in 17 countries in Africa, Asia, the Americas and Europe, which identified the median age of onset for mood disorders as a group as 29–43 years. Prevalence appears relatively low until the early teens, with risk for the onset of depression increasing sharply between the ages of 12 and 16 years and more gradually up to the early 40s, when it begins to decline. Hence, the overall prevalence continues to increase through middle age, with a more gradual increase thereafter.

Survey evidence shows that for common mental disorders as a whole (anxiety, mood and substance-use disorders), onset is at a relatively young age, with narrow age bands for typical ages of onset: half of all lifetime common mental disorders start by the age of 14 years and three-quarters by age 24 years. Although anxiety disorders have a markedly younger age of onset than depression (the median onset age for anxiety disorders is 11 years), these often develop a shared morbidity with depression in later adulthood. This means that for very many adults with depression, their mood problems emerged in early adulthood and any associated anxiety problems are likely to have developed during their adolescence.

Depression course

At least half of all people affected by depression experience more than one episode. Depression relapse is defined as an episode of depression that occurs within 6 months after either response or remission, while recurrence is defined as another depressive episode that occurs after 6 months have elapsed. Recovery from depression is usually understood as a period of full remission lasting at least 8 weeks. A pattern of repeated episodes – including recurrence or relapse – may be the commonest expression of depressive disorder. Several studies have identified rates of recurrence as high as 90% and similarly the NCS-R found that for more than 90% of those people identified with depression, this was a recurrence rather than an initial episode. In terms of the length of time between episodes, this appears variable: once a first episode has occurred, recurrent episodes will usually begin within 5 years of the initial episode, and around 35% of people experience a further episode within 2 years of their first episode.

On average, individuals with a history of depression will have five to nine separate depressive episodes in their lifetime. Risk factors for recurrence are listed in Table 3.2.

There is evidence that few episodes of depression persist beyond 1 year, with several community studies noting that 80% of individuals experiencing an episode had recovered by this time. It is likely that typical episodes of depression experienced in the general population are considerably shorter than has been identified in the patients who are treated by health services, as shorter episodes are obviously less likely to prompt help-seeking. Community studies in the USA indicate mean durations of between 13 and 30 weeks, and median values of around 12 weeks; studies in primary care populations in the USA and France found a mean duration of episode of 12 weeks. For about

TABLE 3.2

Risk factors for depression recurrence*

- An earlier onset of depression (conflicting evidence)
- Greater symptom severity in the first episode
- Specific symptoms: suicidal thoughts and primary sleep disturbance
- Comorbid anxiety disorder, dysthymia and substance-use disorders
- A family history of any mental illness and of affective disorders
- Negative cognitive styles
- High levels of neuroticism
- Stressful life events, both in childhood and particularly in adulthood
- Lack of social support
- Experience of violence and abuse

*Many of these variables are predictors of initial onset as well as of recurrence. Demographic variables such as sex, marital status and socioeconomic status may be important for the initial onset of depression, but do not appear significantly related to the risk of a recurrent course.

Adapted from Burcusa and Iacono, 2007.

20% of people with depression, illness follows a chronic course with persistence of symptoms at diagnostic threshold level for at least 2 years.

In older people. Older people with depression are likely to exhibit a more chronic course, with longer duration of episodes and shorter times to relapse than younger individuals, and around 30% are likely to remain chronically depressed. A meta-analysis of data from 12 primary care and community secondary care studies of depressed patients aged 60 years and over showed that after 2 years, 21% of those who were depressed had died, and among survivors nearly half remained depressed. Subthreshold depression as well as major depression is associated with functional impairment and increased mortality, and together with the risk of suicide – which is highest among older people – underlines the fact that mood disorders are potentially fatal diseases. This more adverse longitudinal trajectory seems to be accounted for by factors such as previous episodes and medical comorbidity (which is explored in Chapter 6). As for other age groups, the number of previous episodes is one of the strongest predictors of relapse and recurrence. Other variables most clearly associated with longer durations of depression episode include poor self-rated health status, depression severity, inadequacy of social support and adverse life events, as well as diagnosed comorbidities.

In younger people. There is conflicting evidence as to whether early onset of depression is predictive of a recurrent course. However, because young adulthood is a critical stage for developing interpersonal relationships, educational qualifications and a career, the incidence of depression in this life stage may consequently have more severe and persistent consequences than for other age groups. Depression in young people is related to greatly increased risks of school exclusion, poor educational achievement and self-harm acts; it is also predictive of teenage childbearing, marital instability, financial adversity and physical and mental ill health in adulthood. The challenge of depression prevention and treatment is important throughout the lifespan, but because of the extent of adversity associated with its early onset, there is a particular need for prevention and early interventions in this age group.

Impact of depression

Disability. The frequency and severity of mental disorders was not fully appreciated until an international study initiated by the World Bank and coordinated by the WHO quantified the extent of disability attributable to particular diseases in the early 1990s. This enterprise – the GBD project (see page 31) – revealed that mental illness accounted for much of the total disability in economically developed and developing countries, with depression identified as the chief cause among this disorder group. Depression is ranked as the third leading cause of burden among all diseases, accounting for 4.4% of the total disability-adjusted life-years (DALYs); it is the leading cause of years lived with disability (YLDs) throughout the world (Table 3.3). (The DALY, developed in 1990 to quantify the burden of diseases, injuries and risk factors, is based on the years of life lost by premature death and YLD.)

The extent of disease burden due to depression is projected to show a rising trend during the coming decade, with it becoming the second leading cause of DALYs lost. Worldwide, it is projected by 2020 to be second only to ischemic heart disease for DALYs lost for both sexes. This is not necessarily related to increased depression incidence or the age of onset becoming younger. Indeed, the evidence for an increased prevalence of this mood disorder in adolescents appears weak when appropriate international population studies are pooled. Changes in global demographics together with the process of transition of population disease burden from acute infectious conditions to non-communicable disorders across the world are the main contributors to this changing picture.

Employment and lost productivity. A significant part of the burden of depression relates to impairment of work function. This affects people with depression and those who experience depression together with medical conditions, where the odds of extended work loss and extended disability are synergistically affected by the disorder combination.

41

TABLE 3.3

The ten leading causes of years lived with disability (YLD) by broad income group, 2001

Cause	YLD (days, millions)	% total YLD
Low- and middle-income countries		
Unipolar depressive disorders	43.22	9.1
Cataracts	28.15	5.9
Hearing loss, adult onset	24.61	5.2
Vision disorders, age-related	15.36	3.2
Osteoarthritis	13.65	2.9
Perinatal conditions	13.52	2.8
Cerebrovascular disease	11.10	2.3
Schizophrenia	10.15	2.1
Alcohol-use disorders	9.81	2.1
Protein-energy malnutrition	9.34	2.0
High-income countries		
Unipolar depressive disorders	8.39	11.8
Alzheimer's and other dementias	6.33	8.9
Hearing loss, adult onset	5.39	7.6
Alcohol-use disorders	3.77	5.3
Osteoarthritis	3.77	5.3
Cerebrovascular disease	3.46	4.9
Chronic obstructive pulmonary disorder	2.86	4.0
Diabetes mellitus	2.25	3.2
Endocrine disorders	1.68	2.4
Vision disorders, age-related	1.53	2.1

Mathers CD, Lopez AD, Murray CJL, eds. The burden of disease and mortality by condition: data, methods, and results for 2001. *Global Burden of Disease and Risk Factors*. New York: OUP, 2006:45–93. Available from www.dcp2.org/pubs/GBD/3/Table/3.12, last accessed 15 July 2011.

People with mental health problems have the lowest employment rate of any disabled group: in the UK nearly 40% of incapacity benefits claimants have mental health problems as their main disability, and mental problems are a secondary factor for another 10% or more. In England, this amounts to over 900 000 adults claiming sickness and disability benefits for mental health conditions. On average, depressed people lose 11 days through time off work every 6 months in comparison with 2 days for people without depression. In the UK, a total of 70 million working days and £4 billion per annum are estimated to be lost because of depression. This does not include the burden of the disorder associated with carers' loss of productivity.

In the USA, the American Productivity Audit (2001–2) examined the extent and costs of productivity lost because of depression, and reached an estimate of $44 billion, in part from work absence, but to a large degree resulting from the effects of depression on work performance.

Social exclusion. The social environment plays a crucial part in determining the quality of people's lives. Participation and social engagement are crucial to the well-being of the individual and have consistently been found to be central to human development and successful aging. Social exclusion is a term that describes marginalization from employment, income and social networks such as one's family, neighborhood and community.

People who are depressed are more likely to experience multiple exclusions, particularly if they are older, on low income or living alone. As well as reducing quality of life this is likely to increase the risk for depression recurrence or persistence, as interpersonal relationships act as a buffer between adverse events and depression. By encouraging continued physical activity and engagement in treatment regimens, social support positively influences function and mood. Conversely, social isolation and loneliness are associated with worsening of depression outcome. These variables are intuitively linked, and research shows loneliness to be a significant risk factor for depression in older people, with the association strongest among people with cognitive impairment. In the UK, a relatively small proportion (7%) of older people report severe loneliness and this proportion, despite concerns about the negative effects of changing family and neighborhood structures, appears to have remained relatively stable over the last 50 years. Vulnerability factors for loneliness include female sex, chronic health problems and marital status (with highest risk among those widowed, then divorced and single compared with married). The all-cause mortality risk of depression in the community-based oldest old (people aged 85 years and older) has been found to be significantly (twofold) increased by the presence of perceived loneliness. The mechanism by which loneliness impacts on health seems to be via a sense of 'giving up' or motivational depletion, which may have a range of negative consequences, such as reduced self-care and mobility, social isolation and poor health behavior. Loneliness resulting from the death of a spouse, or from poor social support and physical illness or disability may be a factor in self-harm and suicide in older people, particularly in older men.

Key points – epidemiology and impact

- Depression is a common mental disorder, affecting around 5% of the population over a 12-month period, with around 20% of people likely to experience depression over the course of their lifetime.
- Women are nearly twice as likely to experience depression than men, and depression more commonly affects people who are divorced or separated, or who have experienced violence or abuse, as well as those experiencing socioeconomic adversity.
- The majority of the disability attributed to mental and neurological disorders in the world is due to depression: nearly 33% as measured by disability-adjusted life-years.
- In high- and middle-income countries, depression is the leading cause of disability and, primarily due to changes in demographic and disease distribution patterns, its contribution to global disability is projected to increase over future decades.
- Depression is related to a range of biological, sociocultural and psychological factors, and though there are strong links between adversity and its onset these events are not necessarily predictive of depression for individuals.
- At least half of all people affected by depression experience more than a single episode, and the risk of recurrence increases with each successive episode.

Key references

Burcusa SL, Iacono WG. Risk for recurrence in depression. *Clin Psychol Rev* 2007;27:959–85.

Costello EJ, Erkanli A, Angold A. Is there an epidemic of child or adolescent depression? *J Child Psychol Psychiatry* 2006;47:1263–71.

Eaton WW, Shao H, Nestadt G et al. Population-based study of first onset and chronicity in major depressive disorder. *Arch Gen Psychiatry* 2008;65:513–20.

Gilchrist G, Gunn J. Observational studies of depression in primary care: what do we know? *BMC Fam Pract* 2007;8:28.

Judd LL, Akiskal HS, Maser JD et al. A prospective 12-year study of subsyndromal and syndromal depressive symptoms in unipolar major depressive disorders. *Arch Gen Psychiatry* 1998;55:694–700.

Kessler RC, Angermeyer M, Anthony JC et al. Lifetime prevalence and age-of-onset distributions of mental disorders in the World Health Organization's World Mental Health Survey Initiative. *World Psychiatry* 2007;6:168–76.

McManus S, Meltzer H, Brugha T et al. *Adult Psychiatric Morbidity in England, 2007: Results of a Household Survey.* Leeds: The NHS Information Centre for Health and Social Care, 2009.

Scott KM, Bruffaerts R, Tsang A et al. Depression–anxiety relationships with chronic physical conditions: results from the World Mental Health Surveys. *J Affect Disord* 2007;103:113–20.

Ustun TB, Ayuso-Mateos JL, Chatterji S et al. Global burden of depressive disorders in the year 2000. *Br J Psychiatry* 2004; 184:386–92.

4 Identification in clinical practice

*My dreams were accompanied by deep seated anxiety and
gloomy melancholy, such as are wholly incommunicable
by words. I seemed every night to descend into chasms and
sunless abysses, depths below depths, from which it seemed
hopeless that I could ever reascend.*

Thomas de Quincey, *Confessions of an
English Opium-Eater*, 1821

Recognizing depression is clearly the essential starting point for any
effective management – whether this is active monitoring, support for
self-help, or more active or health-technology-oriented interventions.
As has been noted, the majority of people with depression will have
initial contact with primary care services and receive ongoing
management from primary care practitioners. In settings where a
well-developed primary care system with a gate-keeping function
exists, such as the UK and Australia, this amounts to around 80%
of people who receive treatment for depression. In the USA, primary
care practitioners manage approximately one-half of adults and nearly
two-thirds of older adults treated for depression.

The findings of studies conducted over several decades and in many
countries reveal that people with depression in primary care have this
condition missed during their consultations – particularly their initial
presentation – relatively often. Although clinicians' problems in
recognizing depression have been most commonly investigated
in primary care settings, this under-recognition has also been noted in
studies of inpatient medical and surgical settings, medical outpatient
clinics, emergency departments and care homes.

Clinician recognition is typically evaluated in these studies by
comparing a diagnosis of depression reached using a validated rating
scale with a specified cut-point or (less commonly) by a standardized
diagnostic interview, with one of the following:

- notation in the patient's clinical record chart of depression as a diagnosis or diagnostic code, or a clear description of depressive symptoms
- referral of the patient to a mental health provider or prescription of antidepressant medication
- clinician-rated depression or probable depression on an encounter form, or score sheet, or in response to face-to-face interview.

The rates of detection by non-psychiatric physicians have generally been found to be low, with measures of sensitivity – the proportion of true cases correctly identified – varying, particularly in relation to the method used by the doctor to recognize depression. A recent systematic review of 36 relevant studies found a summary sensitivity of 36%. Non-psychiatric clinicians' specificity of depression recognition – the proportion of non-cases correctly identified as not being depressed – was much higher, with a summary rate of 84% found in this review.

The inadequate identification of depression is clearly a cause for concern; however, this should be tempered somewhat by the findings of a number of naturalistic studies conducted in several countries indicating that it is milder forms of depression that are most likely to be undetected by non-psychiatrists, and these are more likely to remit spontaneously or they may be less likely to respond to treatments.

Furthermore, most studies of depression recognition in primary care have used a single time point to evaluate recognition, but this may be misleading as clinically significant depression is often detected by primary care providers at later consultations by virtue of the ongoing person-focused care that is the characteristic of primary care. There is evidence that recognition and treatment may occur at a subsequent visit. In one study, approximately half of those with unrecognized depression at baseline had some evidence of recognition at 3 months as indicated by an antidepressant prescription or a mental health referral.

Depression recognition can be examined in relation to patient, clinician/provider and context/system factors (Table 4.1).

TABLE 4.1

Patient, clinician and context variables that influence depression recognition

Patient factors

- Beliefs and attitudes about depression and its treatment
- Stigma and guilt
- Expectation of empathy and non-judgmental response
- Familiarity with communicating emotional issues
- Timing during consultation of broaching psychological concerns (often left till late in consultation)
- Concerns about implications of mental problems being recorded
- Age, sex, ethnicity

Clinician factors

- Knowledge about depression presentation and features
- Attitude concerning depression recognition and treatment
- Communication skills that facilitate patient disclosure and discussion
- Physical symptoms misinterpreted or obscure depressive features

Context

- Duration of consultation
- Incentives for case finding/screening for depression
- Accessible guidelines for best practice in depression assessment
- Access to suitable treatments and referral pathways

Patient factors

Duration of depression. Many people who experience depression do not seek professional help: studies indicate that, at most, only a half of people suffering from major depression in Western economically developed countries seek professional help during the first year of illness. Often people will seek help only after a delay of many years, which is associated with a range of adverse consequences. It appears that young adults are least likely to seek professional help for mental health problems; indeed, people with these early-onset mood and anxiety disorders often wait more than a decade before seeking treatment. This is particularly problematic as these difficulties are likely to have become more seriously impairing, with more severe and long-lasting consequences than if treatment had been sought earlier in the illness course.

Sex. Consultation rates and help-seeking patterns are consistently lower in men than in women, and this is particularly evident for psychological problems and depressive symptoms. Studies from the USA and Australia reveal that this difference in help-seeking behavior is evident in adolescent samples (male:female odds ratio 0.72), and this persists through the lifespan. Although depression is more common among women, the suicide rate for men is nearly four times higher, and their poor use of services prompted one expert to comment 'women seek help – men die'.

Ethnicity and culture may influence depression help-seeking, problem disclosure and expectations in relation to the primary care physician, with differences found in these variables by research studies carried out in Australia and England. Such differences are likely to relate to differences in support networks and remedies that are available or traditionally used (such as folk remedies, religious networks, self-help), as well as misconceptions about depressive symptoms and the role of health services in their treatment. These differences have been found to be particularly pronounced in older people from particular ethnic groups.

Effects of depression. A disinclination to consult or to express features of depression may relate to the reduced motivation, guilt and self-blame, and pessimism (about the outcome of seeking help) that characterize the depressive syndrome. For some patients, disclosure of depression during a consultation may be influenced by concerns about mental health problems being noted in their medical record.

Further barriers to seeking professional help may involve more general negative beliefs and attitudes – including views that particular interventions or professionals are not useful, or that it is better to deal with mood problems by yourself, or negative stereotypes of mental illness. Studies in the USA and Canada reveal that 15–20% of respondents would probably not or definitely not seek treatment if they had serious emotional problems. Almost one-half of survey participants in these countries stated they would be embarrassed if their friends knew about their use of mental health services. In European countries a similar picture emerges: a large-scale study in six countries indicated that almost one-third of the people believed that professional care for serious emotional problems was no better or worse than no help. In regard of these negative views of mental health problems, it appears that older age, a lower education level and less familiarity with mental illness were associated with reduced tolerance of these problems. A survey in the UK revealed a widespread reluctance to consult about emotional problems because of worries about a critical response from the primary care physician.

Studies – mainly Australian – have indicated that peoples' attitudes influence their service use, and in particular may predict seeking professional help for psychological problems, use of antidepressant medication and use of mental health services.

In addition to attitudes and beliefs, people's knowledge about depression can affect their help-seeking, and the literature concerning 'health literacy' – defined as the ability to gain access to, understand and use information in ways which promote and maintain good health – has been extended to encompass such understanding applied to mental health. Studies have shown that members of the general public have limited knowledge about the features and causes of mental disorders, including depression, of the most effective types of help available, and of how to access appropriate help.

Many depressed primary care patients present exclusively with physical symptoms, which they do not attribute to psychological etiologies. Presentation with physical symptoms has been shown to be associated with lower rates of depression recognition and treatment because treating physicians may misattribute varied ill-defined somatic complaints accompanying depression to non-psychological causes.

Initiatives to improve mental health literacy have been conducted in the USA, UK and Europe and, most extensively, in Australia. These have mostly involved mass media health campaigns providing details of the features of depression or other mental health problems, together with the message that depression is common, serious and treatable. Evaluations have indicated that mental health literacy, as well as attitudes and beliefs, can be influenced by such approaches.

Clinician factors

The process of problem formulation and diagnostic reasoning appears to be made up of several stages that involve particular strategies on the part of the clinician, such as attention to initial complaints, identifying symptom patterns, eliciting elements of examination and history, and use of active monitoring/'watchful waiting' or trial treatments. The quality of practitioners' interviewing skills, particularly the appropriate use of open questions, awareness of non-verbal elements of communication, exploration of psychosocial issues and demonstration of empathy, are central to these processes and have, unsurprisingly, been found to be linked to accuracy of detection. Importantly, these aspects of clinical communication have been shown to be modifiable by training interventions.

Awareness of guidance. Clinician knowledge and awareness of relevant clinical guidelines is relevant to correct detection and ongoing management: a UK-wide survey of primary care providers recently identified that just over half of the respondents (58%) were aware of guidelines for the management of depression, and similar findings have been found among physicians in New York, USA.

The attitudes of clinicians are likely to influence their assessment practices and management approaches to this problem type; attitude factors such as interest in psychological problems and a belief in the malleability of such problems to intervention seem likely to be related to an empathic consultation style and responsiveness to depression features in the presentation, while views about depression etiology and the mechanisms related to treatment or problem persistence would be expected to influence the management approaches adopted. While there appears considerable variability in these professional dispositions, attitude surveys (using a specifically devised measure – the Depression Attitude Questionnaire) of primary care physicians have provided some support for these associations. Several studies have shown a link between clinicians' attitudes and their management decisions, and between training courses and primary care physicians' attitudes to the identification and treatment of depression. Examinations of the attitudes of physicians and other health professionals in primary care generally indicate a shared agreement that depression is neither a natural consequence of aging nor a sign of weakness. Overall, clinicians surveyed in a number of European nations felt strongly that depression is amenable to change, and that looking after depressed patients is a rewarding activity. Moreover, primary care physicians throughout European countries are generally opposed to the notion that depressed patients requiring antidepressants are better off with a psychiatrist – with this notion being rejected particularly strongly in the UK.

Presentation with concurrent physical problems increases the difficulties with recognizing depression. In part this is because of competing priorities in the assessment – often patients will voice physical symptoms first, with inadequate opportunity left for exploration of psychological symptoms. Secondly, there is the responsibility on the health professional to ensure that a serious physical illness is not missed or 'masquerading' as depression. Recognition difficulties may also arise because the physical or somatic features of depression – such as insomnia and disturbed sleep, reduced appetite and weight loss, fatigue and psychomotor retardation – may all be related to the medical condition or its treatment. These features may lead the clinician to think that the physical problem is the only reason for the symptoms, which may delay or prevent diagnosis. Despite the confusion that relates to multiple causes for symptoms, it appears that modifications to diagnostic criteria are not an appropriate response to difficulties in this area, and that the somatic symptoms retain their importance in assessing depression in people with physical disease – though a full assessment is always required.

Ethnicity may influence disorder recognition: a study in inner-London general practices found psychological problems among black Africans were less likely to be detected by primary care physicians than those in white or black Caribbean patients. US primary care physicians have been found less likely to detect depression among African-American and Hispanic patients than among whites, particularly if the doctor and patient are of a different race.

Contextual factors

The limitations of consultation duration are a commonly quoted problem affecting the detection of depression. Time constraints are common across regions and nations, with typical primary care consultations being limited to 10–15 minutes; this poses obvious limits on the extent of discussion and exploration of the nature of symptoms, which is of particular relevance in eliciting the elements of history and symptoms pertinent to depression.

Studies of primary care physicians in the UK and Australia have also found that a lack of services to refer people to, problems with waiting time for specialist referrals, and difficulty accessing services are regarded as the main obstacles for primary care depression service delivery. In the USA, primary care clinicians also note the fragmented mental health system and limitations in insurance coverage as barriers to their provision of care.

Improving depression recognition

Several approaches have been identified to improve the quality of depression recognition and management. These have been implemented and evaluated predominantly in primary care, as most people with depression are encountered in this environment. Related innovations and evaluations have covered, for example, emergency departments, general hospitals, care homes and opportunities within perinatal services.

Approaches to implementing clinical practice guidelines

These approaches are part of wider professional development interventions or activities designed to change clinicians' behavior and assist the incorporation of evidence-based knowledge. A broad range of strategies and delivery methods have been used, from the simple provision of printed educational materials, through educational outreach such as in academic detailing, the use of local opinion leaders, targeted audit and feedback, computerized decision-support systems (alerts/reminders) and the local development of evidence-based policies.

A number of reviews of the evidence have been conducted, and findings indicate that printed materials – usually incorporating evidence-based guidelines – appear a necessary, but in themselves insufficient, strategy for improving performance, and similarly passive training activities are associated with limited changes. Multifaceted approaches to clinician education, making use of combinations of educational techniques, are generally better supported by the evidence.

The evidence concerning the impact on patient outcomes of these continuing professional development approaches for depression identification and improved management is limited, and indicates that changes in the organization of care are required. In addition to educational approaches such as teaching events and printed/electronic materials – which can be seen as predisposing elements – approaches to modify the setting or style of care to assist change (enabling elements) and additional follow-up or ongoing prompts to maintain alterations in practice (reinforcing elements) are necessary for sustained changes to occur.

One important element of changed practice involves using validated case-finding measures to enhance accurate detection.

The use of case finding measures. Given the substantial proportion of cases of depression missed in primary care, the use of case-finding tools appears an appealing approach to assist recognition. There are a number of measures that are brief, easy to administer and score, psychometrically robust and acceptable to patients. However, contradictory results are found in published studies of the feedback of

55

such standardized measures to primary care providers. Systematic reviews of randomized controlled trials of the use of screening or case finding in general medical and primary care settings indicate that the routine feedback of instrument results does not increase the recognition rate for depression. Nonetheless, the most recent (2009) US Preventive Services Task Force (USPSTF) review, as well as the analogous Canadian body and the National Institute for Health and Clinical Excellence in England, Wales and Northern Ireland are supportive of the use of case-finding instruments to improve depression care.

There appear to be two main problems with case finding for depression.

- The approach yields a large number of false-positive findings when used within an unselected primary care population.
- Where case finding is used without additional enhancement of the delivery of care, there is no effect on depression outcomes.

Case finding for depression makes sense and is more likely to be associated with clinical benefits when these two difficulties are addressed. When case finding is directed at patient groups with increased risks of depression (and hence a higher prevalence of depression), such as people with long-term physical health problems, the balance of ratios of true- and false-positive cases identified by this approach is markedly different, and this strategy appears justified. An example of this is the adopting (in April 2006) of this method within the National Health Service Quality and Outcomes Framework (QOF), a component of the General Medical Services contract for general practices in England. Practice payments are allocated for the implementation of depression case finding among patients with diabetes and coronary heart disease using a standardized two-question screen.

The finding that implementing screening programs (without further service changes) has minimal effects on improving depression care outcomes may be explained by many screen-detected patients having milder levels of depression than those identified without screening, with the screen-detected patients being be more likely to improve without professional treatment. The way in which the case-finding tools are used also has a bearing, with greater likelihood of benefit in programs where staff other than the primary care physician administer the standardized questionnaire and feed back only the results of screen-positive (high-risk) patients to the clinician. The most important factor relates to enhancing the capacity for depression management. The USPSTF review notes that insufficient treatment, rather than inadequate identification, is the greatest barrier to long-term relief from depression. Although this separation is logically flawed, it is correct that improving identification without ensuring that systems are in place to deliver treatment is inappropriate.

As will be discussed in the following chapter, there are considerable deficits in depression treatment and follow-up, with many people recognized as depressed not provided with appropriate treatment, and of those prescribed antidepressant more than half discontinuing after an inadequate treatment period. The greatest gains for those with major depression are seen in programs where systematic case finding is combined with collaborative care and case management approaches (based on the chronic disease management approach developed by Wagner, Von Korff and others). This involves specific staff roles concerned with assessment, monitoring and coordination between the primary care provider's treatment and any specialty mental health treatment that may be required; further detail of these approaches to depression care are provided in Chapter 5.

Case-finding tools. A large number of case identification tools for depression are available. This has possibly been a source of some confusion for health professionals, in terms of selecting the most appropriate tool and achieving consistency in clinical practice.

Three of the most often used and best validated measures have been recommended for use in UK general practice:

- the depression subscale of the Hospital Anxiety and Depression Scale (HADS)
- the Beck Depression Inventory, 2nd edition (BDI-II)
- the nine-item Patient Health Questionnaire (PHQ-9).

The most widely used of these in UK and US primary care is the PHQ-9. It is a brief empirically validated measure derived from the

Diagnostic and Statistical Manual of Mental Disorders of the American Psychiatric Association, fourth edition (DSM-IV) that has good acceptability in primary care and psychiatric settings to patients and clinicians. It performs well in detecting depression and assessing diagnostic threshold, planning treatment and tracking changes, and it appears to work well in the presence of physical comorbidity. In principle, a higher score on these measures indicates greater severity requiring greater intervention. However, the QOF guidance also recommends that clinicians consider the degree of associated disability, history of depression and patient preference when assessing the need for treatment rather than relying completely on the questionnaire score.

Which patients will most benefit from the use of case-finding tools?
As has been mentioned, the balance of benefits and harms (such as burden on patients and staff, additional activity and expenditure, false-positive screen results) indicates that case-finding tools should not be used with the whole general practice population, but rather with a group of patients who are known to be at increased risk of depression. These standardized measures can play a useful part in the management of some groups of patients, as described below.

- Patients who have chronic medical conditions, such as coronary heart disease, chronic obstructive pulmonary disease and diabetes are at significantly increased risk of depressive episodes, and case-finding tools can play a useful part in such monitoring which may be conducted as part of regular (possibly annual) general reviews.
- Patients who have a history of previous depressive episodes are at higher risk of further episodes, and the use of these measures at regular intervals may assist the prompt recognition of recurrence.
- Patients who are being treated for depression – the measures may play a part in monitoring response to treatment.

The use of the standardized measures as part of a more thorough assessment appears an appropriate approach for these patients. However, it is important to note that initial and ongoing assessments require more than simply applying the measure or counting symptoms.

There is a need to direct attention to any past history of depression and treatment response, current impairment that may be associated with depression, the presence of particular stressors and the availability of social supports.

Alongside the case-finding measures noted above, a further even briefer tool has been found to be useful in primary and general medical practice. A two-question screen requesting a Yes or No response that is presently used in UK primary care (and is sometimes termed the 'Whooley questions') has excellent sensitivity and is recommended in recent NICE guidance for the UK (not Scotland) as the instrument to be used in the assessment of depression in people with chronic physical health problems (sensitivity 0.95 and specificity 0.66 based on seven studies in primary care, chronic physical health, and older populations analysed for NICE guidance) (Table 4.2).

A number of researchers have tried to identify the depressive symptoms that are most predictive of reduced well-being and function, and have attempted to reduce the number of symptoms required to make a diagnosis of depression. Several differing subsets of core symptoms have been identified and tested, and there are indications that these simpler groups of symptoms may be useful. However, the balance of evidence and consensus remains in favor of eliciting and considering the full range of features noted in current diagnostic systems.

TABLE 4.2

Two-question case-finding tool for depression

Question 1: During the past month, have you often been bothered by feeling down, depressed or hopeless?

Question 2: During the past month, have you often been bothered by little interest or pleasure in doing things?

A positive response to either (or both) questions indicates depression is likely. This merits more detailed assessment, which may involve a longer validated tool.

Key points – identification in clinical practice

- Identifying depression is the necessary first stage to enable ongoing monitoring, risk assessment, support, and clinical management; however, many people with depression are not identified in primary care or medical settings.
- A combination of patient, clinician and context-based factors operate to hinder depression identification, but these factors can all be modified to improve the process of condition recognition.
- Interventions to improve recognition that do not incorporate changes to the context and organization of care are likely to have only weak effects on depression outcomes.
- The best evidence indicates the effectiveness of a combined approach involving education for clinicians and patients, systematic use of case-finding tools and organizational changes to improve depression management capacity and sustain practice changes.

Key references

Cabana MD, Rushton JL, Rush AJ. Implementing practice guidelines for depression: applying a new framework to an old problem. *Gen Hosp Psychiatry* 2002;24:35–42.

Gilbody S, Sheldon T, House A. Screening and case-finding instruments for depression: a meta-analysis. *CMAJ* 2008;178: 997–1003.

Maginn S, Boardman AP, Craig TK et al. The detection of psychological problems by General Practitioners— influence of ethnicity and other demographic variables. *Soc Psychiatry Psychiatr Epidemiol* 2004;39:464–71.

Pignone MP, Gaynes BN, Rushton JL et al. Screening for depression in adults: a summary of the evidence for the U.S. Preventive Services Task Force. *Ann Intern Med* 2002;136:765–76.

U.S. Preventive Services Task Force. *Screening for Depression in Adults: Clinical Summary of U.S. Preventive Services Task Force Recommendation. AHRQ Publication No. 10-05143-EF-3.* Rockville: Agency for Healthcare Research and Quality, 2009.

Whooley MA, Avins AL, Miranda J, Browner WS. Case-finding instruments for depression. Two questions are as good as many. *J Gen Intern Med* 1997;12:439–45.

Williams JW, Jr., Pignone M, Ramirez G, Perez Stellato C. Identifying depression in primary care: a literature synthesis of case-finding instruments. *Gen Hosp Psychiatry* 2002;24:225–37.

Talking of constitutional melancholy, he observed, "A man so afflicted, Sir, must divert distressing thoughts, and not combat with them." Boswell: "May not he think them down, Sir?" Johnson: "No, Sir. To attempt to think them down is madness. He should have a lamp constantly burning in his bed chamber during the night, and if wakefully disturbed, take a book, and read, and compose himself to rest. To have the management of the mind is a great art, and it may be attained in a considerable degree by experience and habitual exercise." Boswell: "Should not he provide amusements for himself? Would it not, for instance, be right for him to take a course of chymistry?" Johnson: "Let him take a course of chymistry, or a course of rope-dancing, or a course of any thing to which he is inclined at the time. Let him contrive to have as many retreats for his mind as he can, as many things to which it can fly from itself

James Boswell, The Life of Samuel Johnson, 1791.

Prevention

By far the most research attention has been paid to the treatment of depression, with relatively few studies focusing on approaches to prevent its onset. However, knowledge derived from epidemiological and predictive studies has provided a basis for identifying people who are at increased risk of becoming depressed, and for tackling a range of psychosocial risk factors that are implicated in depression onset.

Preventive strategies may be directed towards:
- the whole population – 'universal prevention'
- selected high-risk groups – 'selective prevention'
- people who have already developed some clinical features but not the full-blown disorder – 'indicated prevention'.

Universal prevention. An area where universal programs appear beneficial is mental health promotion for young people using a whole-school approach. Review findings indicate that such programs can be effective when they are long term (implemented continuously for more than 1 year) and include changes to the school climate, rather than brief class-based mental illness prevention programs.

Universal programs have also sought to improve 'mental health literacy' (public knowledge and beliefs about mental health and mental disorders) to assist the recognition and professional or self-management of problems, and so address the high level of unmet need in this area. Initiatives have been conducted in many countries including the USA, UK, Germany, Norway and, most extensively, Australia. Mostly they have involved mass media health campaigns, such as the Depression Awareness, Recognition and Treatment Program, conducted in the USA in the late 1980s, the National Depression Screening Day also in the USA in the early 1990s, the UK Defeat Depression Campaign organized by the Royal College of Psychiatrists and the Royal College of General Practitioners in the mid 1990s and beyondblue, the national depression initiative in Australia launched in 1999. Also in Australia, a 12-hour training course (Mental Health First Aid [MHFA]) was developed in 2000 to teach skills in recognizing and helping mental health problems such as depression, anxiety and psychosis. This program has been adopted in a number of other countries including Canada, Hong Kong, Finland, England, Wales and Scotland.

Reviews suggest that these programs result in modest improvements in knowledge and attitudes towards depression or suicide (and other mental health problems), but most evaluations have not assessed the durability of these changes. There is also little evidence to date that campaigns or training increase appropriate help-seeking or decrease suicidal behavior.

It may be that there are limits to broad-based community education programs, and that more focused depression-prevention initiatives are required specifically for those who are depressed or suicidal. Although the science of depression prevention is at an early stage, the developing evidence base indicates promising findings, and a recent systematic review has identified good evidence for prevention among at-risk individuals and those with early features. In general, it seems that although universally directed services are a vitally important part of delivering health and social care, the most efficient and effective approaches for depression prevention may be those that target populations at risk rather than broader approaches.

Selective prevention approaches that enhance protective factors using particular psychotherapy approaches appear able to delay the onset of the disorder in a range of at-risk groups. Current evidence indicates that interventions based on cognitive–behavior therapy (CBT) and interpersonal psychotherapy (IPT) are useful approaches. For instance, there are promising findings for the effectiveness of individually delivered support for postnatal women. Both intensive home visits by nurses and health visitors and telephone peer support were found to reduce depression onset when targeted to those at risk. Both antidepressant and problem-solving approaches have been found effective in preventing depression onset in patients with stroke. Other investigations have found reduced depression incidence for patients recently diagnosed with cancer by means of a brief psychological intervention, though effects were limited to those participants at highest risk. Similarly, a CBT intervention for adolescents at risk of depression (having parents with depression together with a personal history of depression or subthreshold symptoms) has shown significant preventive benefits.

Overall, findings from trials conducted in a range of settings indicate that preventive interventions may reduce the incidence of depressive disorders by around 20% compared with treatment-as-usual control groups. The extent of effect means that prevention should play a larger role in the further reduction of the disease burden of depressive disorders. Low participation rates in depression prevention programs have been noted as a problem, but it seems likely that the increased use of communications technologies such as mobile/cell phones and the internet, together with appropriate marketing approaches, will enhance involvement.

Management

The attention applied toward improving recognition of depression in primary care explored in Chapter 4 is encouraging. However, a central problem with innovations to improve detection is that these have not necessarily led to more effective depression management. It appears that many people recognized as depressed are not provided with appropriate treatment, and many of those prescribed antidepressants discontinue these after an inadequate treatment period. These management problems relate to the availability, acceptability and effectiveness of current treatments for depression: although there has been considerable progress over recent decades there remain difficulties and limitations in all these areas.

A central issue in relation to depression management is the heterogeneity of this condition. As has been discussed earlier in the book, depression covers a spectrum of symptoms, and different approaches are appropriate for differing levels and types of presentation. As well as matching different approaches according to severity, there are a number of different treatments that appear equally effective for managing depression, and people receiving the same treatments show a range of differing responses, with 25–30% of people treated showing no improvement with initial treatment. For a substantial proportion of people the clinical benefits of treatment are likely to be incomplete, with many requiring changes and combinations of treatments, and at present around one-third of people achieve only partial remission from symptoms despite treatment.

Types of treatment

There are two main approaches to depression treatment: pharmacotherapy and psychological therapy, and evidence shows that both are effective. Many people prefer psychological treatments, and reviews indicate that dropout rates may be lower for psychological treatment than for drug treatment. There is some evidence that for people with less severe forms of depression, psychological treatments may be more effective than pharmacotherapy. Conversely, antidepressant treatment appears more effective in the treatment of dysthymia and for more severe forms of major depressive disorder.

The forms of psychological therapy best supported by current evidence are CBT, behavioral activation and IPT. In addition, electroconvulsive therapy (ECT) is a well-established treatment with evidence for its effectiveness as a treatment for severe depression; it is generally reserved for those who have not responded to other treatment or when the condition is potentially life-threatening.

Several other approaches have benefits for particular levels or presentations of depression – there is some evidence to support the use of exercise, relaxation training and a range of self-help approaches, as well as befriending for milder levels, while exposure to light is effective for seasonal affective disorder and may be useful as an adjunct to other treatments for non-seasonal depression. Some complementary treatments may be useful – there is evidence that the herbal treatment St John's wort is equivalent to standard antidepressants in mild and moderate depression (although there are important problems that limit its usefulness, which are discussed later in this chapter). The nutritional supplement omega-3 polyunsaturated fatty acids (PUFA) may be useful as an adjunctive treatment for depressive symptoms in bipolar disorder, but the effect is uncertain for unipolar depression. Studies of acupuncture for depression have shown mixed results: compared with sham control there is little evidence of benefit, but there may be an additive benefit when acupuncture is combined with medication.

Validity of findings. The evidence for the effectiveness of all these approaches is derived from randomized controlled trials (RCTs) and systematic reviews of such trials. The RCT is a research method designed to ensure findings are free from bias and confounding influences, but it must be noted that there is a trade-off in determining effect by these methods. The high internal validity of RCTs (freedom from bias) is offset by problems in generalizing the findings to wider populations. Trials are typically conducted over relatively brief time frames compared with treatment in the real world, and the interventions are often delivered and monitored by experts and evaluated in a selected population, the members of which are likely to be free of coexisting conditions and unrepresentative of women, older people, ethnic minorities and the socioeconomically disadvantaged compared with the general population.

Organizational approaches. The effectiveness of individual treatments is clearly important in tackling depression, but much depends on the way that services are organized and enabled to respond to the variability of depression presentation and needs for support within populations. Hence the development and evaluation of ways of delivering services is a key part of depression management. Current evidence suggests that better outcomes could be achieved if primary care practices were better organized to identify and respond to those experiencing depression.

Stepped care is a model of healthcare based on treatments of differing intensity being matched to the needs of the individual, so that the least restrictive approaches (in terms of intensity, inconvenience and cost) are used. Allied with this is the systematic monitoring of progress so that management can be altered (stepped up) if response is inadequate. This way of organizing practice involves standardizing the procedures and indications, and it has been used for the management of diverse conditions from migraine and back pain to diabetes and hypertension. More recently it has been advocated for mental health problems such as anxiety, bulimia and depression. A stepped care framework for providing identification and treatment options appropriate to the differing needs of people with depression has been adopted in the UK and is integral to systems for depression care developed in health maintenance organizations in the USA. The stepped care model advocated in the guidance for depression developed by the National Institute for Health and Clinical Excellence (NICE) for use in the National Health Service in England, Wales and Northern Ireland is shown in Table 5.1. The subsequent sections of this chapter will review treatment approaches for depression with reference to this stepped approach.

Chronic care models. Many of the central elements of chronic care models (Table 5.2) have been integrated in the management of depression in adults and older people, and also for people with depression and coexisting physical illnesses. Much of the evaluation of

67

TABLE 5.1

The stepped care model recommended by the National Institute for Health and Clinical Excellence (2009)

Step	Focus of management	Types of intervention
1	Recognition of depression	• Assessment • Referral • Active monitoring • Education and support
2	Treatment of mild to moderate depression	• Medication • Low-intensity psychosocial interventions • Referral to other supports
3	Treatment of: • mild to moderate depression with poor response to interventions • moderate and severe depression	• Medication • High-intensity psychological therapy • Combined treatments • Referral to other supports
4	Treatment of: • severe or complicated depression • severe self-neglect • significant suicide risk	• Medication • High-intensity psychological therapy • Combined treatments • Multiprofessional care • Electroconvulsive therapy • Inpatient care

these approaches has been conducted in the USA, but some evidence for effectiveness has also emerged from studies in the UK and Europe.

Enhanced care packages. It appears that the use of an 'enhanced care' package including stepped care, case management and collaborative care is beneficial and cost-effective for those experiencing moderate-to-severe major depression. An important ingredient of this care appears to be case management – a specific care-coordinator role, usually carried out by a nurse, social worker or psychologist. This appears to be beneficial because it enables more responsive and proactive treatment, allows consistent psychosocial support and assists with understanding and adhering to treatments, as well as developing

TABLE 5.2

Central elements of chronic care models

- The use of clinical information systems to enable systematic and proactive follow-up and review
- Systematic case identification and risk stratification
- Support for self-care, such as education, problem-solving, goal-setting and peer support
- Use of evidence-based guidelines, including protocols, disease-management templates and practitioner education
- Clear arrangements for shared care between primary and specialist providers
- An emphasis on the role of community resources such as voluntary sector organizations
- The use of a case manager to coordinate care

self-management. Telephone as well as face-to-face support is commonly used, and outcomes are routinely measured – using instruments such as the Patient Health Questionnaire (PHQ-9).

Subclinical and mild to moderate depression

Many presentations of depressive symptoms are likely to be relatively short lived and uncomplicated: spontaneous remission and placebo response are relatively common, with around 30% of people improving without active treatment or showing response to inactive management approaches. These presentations do not require formal professional treatment. However, this does not equate to such episodes being insignificant as they may be a precursor to a more serious disorder, and in the early stages of a depressive episode there are limited indicators that may reliably guide the individual or clinician to the likely course.

For this reason, the most appropriate approaches for initial depression onset and for mild depression involve establishing a therapeutic relationship (use of active listening, non-judgmental approach, ensuring confidentiality) and providing simple psychoeducation, while actively monitoring symptoms ('watchful waiting'). If a depressive episode of mild to moderate severity develops, the first options for treatment should include low-intensity interventions such as guided self-help, activity scheduling, brief psychological interventions, supervised exercise programs and computerized CBT (CCBT).

Guided self-help involves the use of written materials, such as books or self-help manuals (other media may be used but the majority of programs are in book form) that provide information about depression, symptom management, condition monitoring and strategies to improve mood and function. These materials are based on evidence, usually a cognitive–behavioral approach, and are most commonly individually delivered though they may also be conducted in a group. Typically, a health professional introduces and explains the materials and monitors and reviews the treatment outcome via limited further contacts. These may be face-to-face, by telephone or by email. A recent systematic review (conducted for the NICE guidance on depression in adults) indicated this approach to be effective in reducing depression scores in comparison with waiting list controls or treatment as usual. Another review that combined trials of book-, computer- and internet-facilitated interventions and examined outcomes among people with depression and anxiety disorders concluded that guided self-help and face-to-face treatments for these conditions have comparable effects.

Exercise. Although around 60 controlled evaluations of the effect of exercise for depression have been conducted, the evidence is inconclusive, primarily because of weaknesses in the design of many of the studies. A range of different types of physical activity have been examined including aerobic (training of cardiorespiratory capacity) and non-aerobic (such as muscular strength or endurance training) exercise, ranging from water aerobics, ballroom dancing, jogging, running, walking and Qigong (a Chinese system of prescribed physical exercises involving breathing, coordination and relaxation and performed in a meditative state).

Overall, physical exercise seems to improve depressive symptoms in people with a diagnosis of dysthymia or mild or moderate depression, but the extent of the effect diminishes to borderline significance when evidence from only the most robust trials is used. Observational studies commonly find that people self-report that they use exercise to avoid depressive symptoms and prevent relapse. Robust evidence to support these claims is currently lacking.

While the evidence indicates that exercise is superior to waiting-list or no-treatment controls, findings are inconclusive concerning equivalence or superiority to either antidepressants or psychological therapy. It appears that discontinuation rates are lower for exercise than antidepressants, though the rate of drop-out from exercise programs may be substantial.

Important questions remain concerning the most effective type, frequency and duration of exercise: the studies that comprise the evidence base involve a wide range of types of physical activity conducted for periods from 10 days to 16 weeks, conducted indoors and outdoors, and including both individual and group approaches and supervised and unsupervised delivery. Reviewers have found that both insufficient data and inadequately reported intervention details make it difficult to identify the characteristics of exercise most likely to be associated with benefit. It appears likely that mixed rather than purely aerobic exercise is most effective, and that forms with higher intensity and longer duration are most likely to be beneficial, although this is based on very limited data.

Not only does physical exercise appear to be beneficial for depression, it has the important additional advantage of delivering health gains in other areas. Although encouragement of any increase in physical activity is likely to be useful for all people with depression, current evidence indicates that a regular program of activity is necessary for maintenance of effects. The most recent (2009) NICE guidance notes that a typical intervention is likely to involve supervised exercise for 45 minutes to 1 hour, undertaken two to three times each week over 10 to 14 weeks.

Given the lack of evidence of superiority of particular kinds of physical activity or modes of delivery, it seems sound to encourage people with depression to choose forms of exercise they most enjoy, as this is likely to maximize continuation in the long term.

71

There is some additional weak evidence (11 trials are included in a recent 2009 Cochrane review) that indicates exercise may be effective in reducing depression and anxiety in children and adolescents.

A systematic review of yoga found the intervention potentially useful for adults with depression, although the conclusions were limited by the poor quality of the studies.

Problem-solving therapy (PST) is a discrete structured time-limited psychological intervention defined as a goal-oriented collaborative and active process that involves identifying and prioritizing particular problems from among the person's current difficulties. It aims to help people to use their own skills and resources to improve their functioning. The treatment usually consists of six sessions, the first of which lasts 1 hour, with subsequent sessions half hourly. It is based on establishing a link between current problems and psychological functioning, with success in solving and establishing control over these problems associated with improvement in depressive symptoms.

Important strengths of this approach are its brevity, accessibility and feasibility for delivery by a range of professionals and paraprofessionals within primary care. Several studies have supported the effectiveness of problem-solving treatment in primary care, but the extent and robustness of the evidence are limited. A recent trial of problem-solving treatment delivered by community mental health nurses compared with usual physician-led primary care found no significant differences in effectiveness. A systematic review of psychosocial interventions delivered in primary care by primary care physicians indicated that this approach was the most promising.

Relaxation training. A variety of techniques are available for inducing relaxation, including progressive muscle relaxation, relaxation imagery, autogenic training and methods adapted from yoga and meditation. These approaches are generally well received by clients, with low drop-out rates evident in studies. One 2008 systematic review (which included 11 trials in the meta-analysis) indicated that relaxation training was more effective at reducing self-rated depressive symptoms than waiting-list, no-treatment or minimal-treatment controls, although outcome measurement by clinician-rated depressive symptoms provided inconclusive differences. Relaxation appears less effective than established psychotherapies such as CBT, but because it requires only brief training it may be useful as an initial element in a stepped care approach. It may, however, be better practice to invest in approaches with stronger evidence of effect such as guided self-help and computer- or internet-delivered treatments.

Sleep hygiene. Disturbed sleep is one of the most common symptoms of depression, occurring in around three-quarters of episodes; it is also a common prodromal feature of depression, preceding depressive episodes in about 40% of cases. It causes subjective distress and can aggravate other symptoms of depression. Assisting people with the sleep difficulties that form a part of the spectrum of depressive features is an important part of initial intervention. 'Sleep hygiene' relates to the promotion of sleep that is appropriately timed and effective. Good sleep hygiene involves adhering to all elements of sleep hygiene guidance (Table 5.3), with particular emphasis on the importance of getting up at the same time each day.

Psychological approaches using the computer and internet. One of the main barriers to patients receiving appropriate psychological treatments, such as CBT or PST, is a shortage of clinicians who can deliver them. Additionally, there may be problems for individuals scheduling appointments with family, work or carer commitments. Internet-based CBT programs, such as MoodGYM and the Sadness Program in Australia, make use of the same techniques as face-to-face therapy but are delivered in a more accessible and cost-effective way via a website. Evaluations of a range of computer- and internet-based CBT programs indicate significant improvements in the symptoms of depression compared with control patients. There is some indication that improvements in symptoms are maintained over time (up to 12 months). The use of such innovations in delivery may be particularly useful in rural and remote settings where access to clinicians may be limited.

TABLE 5.3

Sleep hygiene activities for improving sleep quality

- A clear routine is important, and a consistent waking time is more important than bedtime: get up at the same time each day, 7 days a week

- If you are not asleep after about 20 minutes, go to another room and do something relaxing, such as listening to soothing music, before returning to bed

- Keep your bedroom dark, reducing stimulation such as noise; keep the room cooler rather than warmer

- Avoid stimulating activity such as heated discussions or work before going to sleep

- A regular exercise program helps sleep, but not in the hours prior to bedtime

- Avoid caffeine (coffee, tea, cola drinks) within 7 hours of bedtime

- Avoid alcohol in the evening, as it can reduce the quality of sleep or make you wake in the night

- A light carbohydrate snack before bed may be helpful

- Avoid naps; sleep should be reserved for bedtime

- A wind-down routine before going to bed (e.g. reading, having a warm bath or listening to music) can make it easier to sleep

Moderate and moderate-to-severe major depression

The main options for the treatment of moderate and severe depressions involve pharmacological and psychological interventions. Treatment choice depends on judgments of severity, previous response to interventions and the person's preferences. Both pharmacological and psychological interventions increase response and remission to a similar extent compared with controls, and trials indicate an improvement for around two-thirds of those in any actively treated group. Lower rates of dropout from treatment are usually seen for psychological interventions.

Pharmacological treatments. In the early 1950s the first antidepressant drugs were developed: the monoamine oxidase inhibitors (MAOIs) and, later, the tricyclic antidepressants (TCAs). These drugs act by enhancement of neurotransmission of serotonin and norepinephrine (noradrenaline), as well as other neurotransmitters. Problematically, TCAs have marked anticholinergic and antihistamine effects, and are toxic in overdose, while MAOIs have interactions with foods containing tyramine (red wines, cheese, liver, yeast extract) that cause a potentially fatal hypertensive reaction. For these reasons MAOIs are not commonly used, and are rarely prescribed in primary care; TCAs are more frequently used in primary and secondary care but because of their interactions and side effects are contraindicated in a number of physical illnesses, in particular cardiac disease. They are not recommended as a first-line treatment because of their side effects and interactions together with their toxicity: importantly, TCAs should be avoided where there appears a risk of suicide because (except for lofepramine) they are associated with greatest risk in overdose.

In the late 1980s more selective drugs were developed, with a primary focus of activity on the serotonergic system giving rise to the selective serotonin reuptake inhibitors (SSRIs). Drugs targeting the noradrenergic systems were also developed and antidepressants that combine action on both systems are now also available.

Some recent reviews have questioned the extent of benefit of antidepressants, and there seems little doubt that, as in many other areas of medical treatment, publication bias (wherein studies with positive findings are most likely to be published) has led to an inflated view of antidepressant effectiveness. It also appears that pharmaceutical industry sponsorship of studies is linked to biases in the reporting of findings. But, despite these important limitations, the majority of well-conducted meta-analyses provide evidence of the effectiveness of antidepressants for moderate and severe major depression, as well as for persistent subthreshold or mild depression (dysthymia). It seems, in general, that the more severe the symptoms, the greater the benefit of antidepressant treatment. The findings from a very large number of studies show that, for people with depression of at least moderate severity, around 20% will improve without any treatment and 30% will respond to placebo treatment, while up to 50% will respond to antidepressant treatment.

In the USA, 28 antidepressant medications approved by the Food and Drug Administration (FDA) are noted in current National Institute of Mental Health (NIMH) literature, while 27 are listed in the current British National Formulary (BNF). This diversity of treatment is not necessarily associated with increased effectiveness: there are relatively modest differences between the individual drugs or classes of drug. The main advantage from developments in antidepressants is in terms of tolerability and adverse effects, and notably the risk of harm in overdose.

The SSRIs are far safer in overdose than TCAs, and are generally better tolerated than antidepressants from other classes. Systematic reviews conducted for recent clinical guidelines indicate that, for people with depression, including those with comorbid physical illness, SSRIs are an appropriate first-line treatment. Among this class of drugs the NICE guideline for depression and chronic physical illnesses (2009) notes that sertraline and citalopram appear to have the lowest interaction potential and may be protective of cardiac events, with evidence of benefits in reducing the risk of cardiac morbidity and mortality among people both with and without pre-existing ischemic heart disease.

Another recent systematic review has compared the relative effects of 12 antidepressants (SSRIs and newer third-generation antidepressants) and found sertraline and escitalopram (the S-stereoisomer of citalopram) to have the most favorable balance between efficacy and acceptability.

New antidepressants are being researched and developed that better enhance neurotransmission and influence allied mechanisms; one such development is an antidepressant (agomelatine) that acts at melatonin receptors in addition to serotonin receptors. This novel mode of action appears to be associated with effects of comparable size with those of other antidepressants, but provides greater improvement in sleep and fewer side effects than comparator medications.

For people whose symptoms respond poorly to antidepressants, reviewing side effects, treatment preferences and adherence is warranted. Many people discontinue their antidepressant treatment before the recommended adequate treatment period (6 months continuation after symptom remission): findings from the USA indicate that 42% of patients stop taking antidepressants within the first month of prescribing, and 72% within the first 3 months. Communication between clinician and patient about treatment concerns (such as worries that antidepressants may be addictive), risk and experience of side effects, and likelihood of relapse are helpful in facilitating treatment adherence.

Dose alteration may be beneficial, or switching to another medication, with choice guided by such considerations as previous treatment history and the potential of the drug to cause side effects. Switching between antidepressants because of poor response to initial treatment is more likely to be needed for people with more chronic depression and more coexisting health problems. If there is poor response to these strategies, augmentation with another psychotropic drug such as lithium, an antipsychotic or another antidepressant may be considered. This is usually undertaken in consultation with a consultant psychiatrist or within a specialist mental health service.

Adverse effects of antidepressants. All antidepressants may cause side effects, but TCAs are associated with a greater burden of anticholinergic side effects such as dry mouth, blurred vision and related cardiovascular effects such as hypotension, tachycardia and QT_c prolongation; they also cause sedation and drowsiness. The SSRIs are associated with headache and gastrointestinal (GI) symptoms, and are more likely to cause sexual dysfunction and GI bleeds.

Cardiovascular disease and depression are strongly associated, and a number of antidepressants can increase the risk of adverse events in this patient group. TCAs are particularly noted for their cardiotoxicity, while the SSRIs do not appear to be linked to increased risks for cadiovascular events and may exert a protective effect.

Bleeding effects. SSRIs affect platelet aggregation and vasoconstriction leading to increased bleeding times: the use of these antidepressants for people with risk factors for GI hemorrhage, or who are concurrently taking non-steroidal anti-inflammatory drugs (NSAIDs) should be avoided, and special monitoring and the use of gastroprotective agents is required where such treatments cannot be avoided.

Suicidal ideas and acts may be increased in the early stages of antidepressant treatment. This is a small but very important effect that is most evident in children and adolescents, but remains for those aged below 25 years. Careful consideration of treatment options and close monitoring of people at risk of suicide is essential. If antidepressants are used with people judged to be at risk of suicide, frequent monitoring and reviews are essential. Direct contact is recommended within 1 week of prescribing and thereafter at regular intervals depending on the level of risk and response to treatment. Telephone reviews may usefully supplement direct contacts. The quantity and toxicity of the prescribed antidepressant is an important consideration, and judgment of risk by assessing depression features, conducting a comprehensive suicide risk assessment (Table 5.4), and consideration of social situation and supports are all key factors in deciding whether to involve specialist mental health services.

Antidepressant discontinuation symptoms may occur when stopping treatment; this can affect one-third of people. Although this response may occur with any antidepressant, it is most commonly linked to paroxetine, venlafaxine and amitriptyline. Typical features are sweating, irritability, headache, dizziness, nausea and symptoms that are sometimes indistinguishable from depression itself. To avoid discontinuation symptoms, antidepressants should be withdrawn slowly. Although some people experience severe and prolonged discontinuation symptoms, especially when the antidepressant has been stopped abruptly, symptoms are usually mild and self-limiting if withdrawal is done slowly. There is no evidence of tolerance or cravings developing for antidepressants such as those commonly seen with drugs such as the benzodiazepines. The risk of these withdrawal features should be part of the discussion and explanation in the initial treatment planning and ongoing monitoring with the patient. When antidepressants are stopped, this should be by gradual dose reduction over a 4-week period. If there is a history of discontinuation symptoms, a longer timeframe may be required and should be negotiated with the patient.

TABLE 5.4

Suicide risk assessment*

- Consider the patient in light of known risk factors for suicide (see page 105)
  - male sex
  - diagnosable mental disorder
  - previous suicide attempts/self-harm
  - significant life events
  - substance misuse
  - unemployment
- Assess current mental state and clarify any diagnosis (depression, substance misuse and schizophrenia are associated with particular risk)
- Assess any physical health difficulties
- Assess for current suicide intent in the context of empathic, sensitive and reassuring communication
  - it is useful to 'build up' questions in a progressive way: ask if feeling *pessimistic*, and if so ask specifically about plans for the future and *hopelessness*
  - ask if any *thoughts* of suicide, if so any *intentions* or *plans*
  - use direct questions: most people will reveal suicidal thoughts and there is evidence that suicidal patients are often relieved to be asked about their suicidal intentions
  - ask if any previous acts or attempts; if there has been a recent act, what was the intention and means, and what was the patient's expectation of the lethality of the method.
- Never agree to keep suicidal threats or plans confidential
- Identify any precipitating factors
- Determine any support networks available to the patient
- Reach a judgment of the level of risk based on assessment, and devise a shared plan that is appropriate to this risk level, and that relates to precipitants and supports
- If you are uncertain or concerned, consult with colleagues
- If the patient appears to have a high suicide risk, seek advice from mental health specialists and refer urgently

* Judgment of risk is based on a review of known risk factors, current intentions, prior history of suicidal thoughts and acts, and current emotional state.

Serotonin syndrome is a drug toxicity reaction that involves shivering, sweating, agitation, confusion, delirium, changes in blood pressure, pyrexia and myoclonus. Onset may be rapid, symptoms may range from mild to severe, and the condition may be fatal. It is caused most usually by medicine combinations that increase synaptic serotonin. Management involves the immediate cessation of precipitating medicines and the use of serotonin antagonists and benzodiazepines where necessary.

Antidepressant continuation. For those who meet the criteria for an episode of major depression, antidepressant treatment should be continued for at least 6 months after the remission of an episode of depression (and for 12 months in older people), as this greatly reduces the risk of relapse. Stopping antidepressant treatment should involve a discussion between the patient and clinician, and this review should consider the possible need for continued treatment. There is consistent evidence that continuing treatment with antidepressants reduces the risks of depression relapse, and for patients who are at high risk of recurrence, prescribing should continue for at least 2 years.

People with risk of relapse for whom longer-term treatment must be considered include those who have experienced two or more recent episodes of depression, or who have residual symptoms or prolonged or severe episodes. The dose of medication for this maintenance should be at the same level as the acute treatment. Some psychological treatments have promising effects in the prevention of relapse and recurrence, even after the discontinuation of antidepressants.

Other biological treatments

St John's wort (*Hypericum perforatum*) extracts have been used for centuries as a depression treatment in Germany and have become popular in many other countries, including the UK. It has similar effectiveness to standard antidepressants for mild and moderate depression, and has less frequent and less serious side effects. However, inconsistencies in preparations and uncertainties about dose limit its usefulness, and there are serious interactions with frequently used drugs such as oral contraceptives, anticonvulsants and anticoagulants.

Transcranial magnetic stimulation is a non-invasive process that uses an electromagnetic coil to excite or inhibit cortical areas of the brain. It has been used for physiological studies and as a treatment for depression. Although there are some promising trial findings, to date systematic review of the evidence suggests no strong evidence for benefit.

Nutrition, diet and dietary supplements. Omega-3 polyunsaturated fatty acids (PUFA) (predominantly found in oily fish and widely available as a nutritional supplement) form a part of the Mediterranean diet and may be beneficial for a number of medical conditions. Studies have examined effects for depression, but despite promising initial findings derived from observational studies, the evidence for effect in depression is weak, with recent trials failing to show a significant effect for this either as an augmentation strategy or as a treatment.

5-Hydroxytryptophan (5-HTP) and tryptophan are dietary supplements regarded as natural alternatives to antidepressants. Studies suggest they are better than placebo at alleviating depression, but they may pose a risk for a potentially fatal condition (eosinophilia–myalgia syndrome). This, allied with the fact that their mode of action is the same as effective and well-tolerated antidepressants, makes their usefulness very limited.

Psychological treatments. Many people may prefer a non-drug treatment for depression or one that is consistent with their own view of their problem. Psychological treatments have a lengthy history in the treatment of depression. There are many approaches used to treat depression; the six main treatment types are described in the next subsections.

There is good evidence that psychological therapies are beneficial for depression, and several reviews have found that there are only modest differences between these treatment types. But those systematic reviews with the most rigorously applied criteria have consistently identified differences, with approaches that are directive and teach new skills (IPT, CBT, behavioral activation [BA] and mindfulness-based cognitive therapy [MBCT]) appearing to be more effective than counseling and psychodynamic therapy.

These psychological treatments are effective in both specialist and primary care settings, although one recent review identified lower effects in primary care and suggested selection for therapy by systematic screening rather than referral by the primary care physician was responsible for this lower effect size.

Alongside the widely voiced concerns about the role of pharmaceutical companies, with their drive for profits, in promoting and emphasizing the benefits of antidepressants, there has been recent re-evaluation of the effects of psychological therapy for adult depression, indicating that both publication bias and limitations in quality selection of studies for meta-analysis have caused the effectiveness of psychological treatments to be overestimated. Their effects are significant, and clinically important, but seem likely to be smaller than has been previously assumed.

Psychodynamic and psychoanalytic approaches to therapy originate from the work of Freud in the early 20th century and involve exploring conscious and unconscious conflicts and examining how these are played out in relationships, including the relationship between therapist and client. As such they are non-directive approaches. These therapies are often long term, but treatments for depression that have been evaluated are generally short-term psychodynamic psychotherapies conducted over 10 to 30 sessions.

Counseling refers to a range of interventions, often delivered in primary care and by voluntary sector organizations, that are based on the humanistic psychology model and work of Carl Rogers in the 1950s and 60s. Contemporary counseling, although rooted in these theories, draws on a variety of other sources such as behavioral, psychodynamic and cognitive models.

Behavioral treatments for depression are based on learning theory, and were initially developed in the 1950s. The BA approach involves encouraging the person to alter patterns of negative reinforcement by scheduling pleasurable activities, particularly with others, and to extend activities to encompass more rewarding behaviors. This has been part of CBT, but over the past decade there has been increased interest and application of BA as a therapy in its own right.

CBT originated from the work of Aaron Beck in the 1950s, being formalized into a depression treatment in the late 1970s. It has subsequently been further refined and developed for various other conditions. The key focus is on the ways of thinking that are characteristic of depression and reflect underlying negative beliefs. CBT helps the person to recognize and modify negative thinking through structured collaborative work in therapy sessions and homework assignments. It can be delivered at an individual or group level.

Interpersonal psychotherapy is a more recent therapy, developed for depression treatment in the 1980s, and focusing on current personal relationships and their effects on mood.

MBCT has been developed from mindfulness-based stress reduction, which has been effective for helping patients cope with symptoms related to a broad range of chronic illnesses. It is derived from the Eastern meditative practice of mindfulness, and delivered as an 8-week group program with a further four follow-up sessions in the year after therapy.

Residual symptoms, chronic depression and combination treatments

For a large group of people, remission from depression is partial, with features persisting after initial treatments. This limits function and quality of life and is an indicator of greater risk of relapse. Poor treatment response is more likely for people with coexisting medical problems and with concurrent mental health problems such as anxiety disorders or substance misuse, negative social circumstances and for those whose depression is more chronic. Ongoing treatment steps are successful in improving remission rates – a large-scale study in the USA (the STAR-D study) has shown that around two-thirds of people achieve remission with up to four successive treatments.

When response to antidepressant treatment is suboptimal, switching to CBT is likely to achieve outcomes as good as those achieved by changing to a different antidepressant, and this option may be better tolerated. It is also clear that when response to single treatment types is suboptimal, a combination of antidepressants and CBT is more effective than either treatment alone. MBCT also appears to be a useful adjunct to antidepressant treatment, as a well as a relapse prevention approach in its own right.

As well as for chronic and treatment-resistant depressions, combinations of psychological therapy and antidepressants are also indicated for depression at the most serious end of the severity spectrum. SSRIs together with CBT are currently the best-evaluated approach.

Key points – prevention and management

- The treatment rather than the prevention of depression has dominated agendas to date. However, better understanding of depression risk factors is enabling the emergence and evaluation of preventive approaches, and there are indications that incidence may be substantially reduced by these methods.
- Depression is complex, and understanding and helping requires a sensitive weighing up of the many factors that are relevant to the individuals and families affected.
- There are a range of treatments that may be effective for depression, and matching management intensity to the level of depression severity – termed 'stepped care' – is a widely adopted framework for care.
- For milder forms of depression, self-help, relaxation, sleep hygiene, exercise and problem-solving therapy are likely to be effective; for moderate to severe depression, antidepressants or a structured psychological treatment (cognitive–behavior therapy [CBT]) is indicated; combined antidepressants and psychological therapy may be most appropriate for severe depression.
- Selective serotonin reuptake inhibitor (SSRI) antidepressants are the first-choice medication – but prior treatment history, medical history and drug interactions are key considerations in treatment selection.

Key references

Bodenheimer T, Wagner EH, Grumbach K. Improving primary care for patients with chronic illness: the chronic care model, part 2. *JAMA* 2002;288:1909–14.

Cuijpers P, Donker T, van Straten A et al. Is guided self-help as effective as face-to-face psychotherapy for depression and anxiety disorders? A systematic review and meta-analysis of comparative outcome studies. *Psychol Med* 2010:1–15.

Cuijpers P, van Straten A, Schuurmans J et al. Psychotherapy for chronic major depression and dysthymia: a meta-analysis. *Clin Psychol Rev* 2010;30:51–62.

Cuijpers P, van Straten A, Smit F et al. Preventing the onset of depressive disorders: a meta-analytic review of psychological interventions. *Am J Psychiatry* 2008;165:1272–80.

Cuijpers P, van Straten A, van Oppen P, Andersson G. Are psychological and pharmacologic interventions equally effective in the treatment of adult depressive disorders? A meta-analysis of comparative studies. *J Clin Psychiatry* 2008;69:1675–85; quiz 839–41.

Geddes JR, Carney SM, Davies C et al. Relapse prevention with antidepressant drug treatment in depressive disorders: a systematic review. *Lancet* 2003;361:653–61.

Gellatly J, Bower P, Hennessy S et al. What makes self-help interventions effective in the management of depressive symptoms? Meta-analysis and meta-regression. *Psychol Med* 2007;37:1217–28.

Haddad PM, Anderson IM Recognising and managing antidepressant discontinuation symptoms. *Adv Psychiatr Treat* 2007;13:447–57.

Jorm AF, Morgan AJ, Hetrick SE. Relaxation for depression. *Cochrane Database Syst Rev* 2008:CD007142.

Mental Health First Aid. Information available from www.mhfa.com.au, last accessed 15 July 2011.

National Institute for Health and Clinical Excellence. *Depression: the Treatment and Management of Depression in Adults (Updated Edition) (Clinical Guideline 90).* London: National Institute for Health and Clinical Excellence, 2009.

Spek V, Cuijpers P, Nyklicek I et al. Internet-based cognitive behaviour therapy for symptoms of depression and anxiety: a meta-analysis. *Psychol Med* 2007;37:319–28.

Wagner EH. Chronic disease care. *BMJ* 2004;328:177–8.

I have got so low that I have asked to be hospitalised and for deep narcosis (sleep). I cannot stand being awake. The pain is too much... Something has happened to me, this vital spark has stopped burning – I go to a dinner table now and I don't say a word, just sit there like a dodo. Normally I am the centre of attention, keep the conversation going – so that is depressing in itself. It's like another person taking over, very strange. The most important thing I say is 'good evening' and then I go quiet

Spike Milligan, *Depression and How to Survive It* (Milligan & Clare), 1994

Mental and physical health are closely connected: there is consistent evidence from cross-sectional studies that depression and other mental health problems, such as anxiety or substance misuse, are more common in people suffering from communicable and non-communicable diseases. Large-scale community studies in Canada (Canadian Community Health Survey, 2000/1; National Population Health Survey [conducted every 2 years since 1994]), the USA (Medical Outcomes Study, 1987–9) and elsewhere, with samples of between 11 000 and over 100 000 people, show that this association remains after controlling for such factors as age, sex and social support. The relationship between depression and medical illness appears strongest for conditions that are painful and disabling, prompting the possibility that these attributes of medical illness are the influential factors for the association.

The prevalence of depression among a range of medically ill populations has been widely investigated, and this research shows rates of depression two- to threefold higher than among comparable groups of people not experiencing such diseases (Table 6.1). Alternatively, studies that have examined the existence of medical conditions among people with depression have found this to be very common: one study in 14 regional centers in the USA involving more than 2500 outpatients with depression found that 50% had disabling general medical conditions.

The presence of depression together with medical illness has important implications for the individual, their carers and for health services and society. This combination has complex and extensive effects, involving negative impact on illness course and disability, the uptake of treatments, risk of complications and death rates. It also complicates the way in which people seek help for their problems, and it can interfere with the recognition of their problems by clinicians. The extent of these adverse effects is particularly clear for cardiovascular disease: depression is a well-recognized risk factor for new onset and for recurrences of established disease; and among patients with heart disease the relative risk of subsequent cardiac mortality is increased threefold in those with depression compared with cardiac patients who are not depressed. This increased risk remains after adjusting for confounding factors.

Depression combined with medical illness causes greater disability than these conditions in isolation, and the extent of lost productivity and healthcare use is greatly increased when these conditions exist together. A recent survey of nearly a quarter of a million adults from 60 countries showed that people with comorbid depression reported worse overall health than those with physical illnesses (such as asthma, diabetes or cardiovascular disease) alone. This has led the WHO to highlight the negative effects of depression on physical illnesses among one of its ten most important global public health statistics for 2007.

Pathways and directions

The association between depression and physical health problems could operate through several different pathways.

- Depression may predict and be a risk factor in the development of medical illness.
- Medical illness may predict and play a causal influence in the development of depression.
- The development of both depression and medical illness may relate to a shared cause or risk factor.
- Depression may be related to the effects of medical illness treatment

TABLE 6.1

Comorbidity of depression and selected long-term conditions

Study/review	Survey setting (sample size)	Depression prevalence*
Parkinson's disease		
Weintraub et al. (2006)	Outpatients (n = 148)	22%
Stroke		
Robinson (2003), review	18 inpatient studies (n = 1865)	36% (19% major, 19% minor)
	15 outpatient studies (n = 1693)	33% (23% major, 15% minor)
	4 community studies (n = 1083)	32% (14% major, 9% minor)
COPD		
Wagena et al. (2005)	Occupational cohort (n = 4468/4520)	14%
van Ede et al. (1999), review	9 studies, largely outpatient (n = 771)	7–29% (dependent on diagnostic method)
CHD		
Lett et al. (2004), review	5 studies, hospitalized and outpatient (n = 1059)	14–23% (major)
Rudisch and Nemeroff (2003), review	5 studies, hospitalized and outpatient (n = 880)	17–23% (major)
Diabetes[†]		
Anderson et al. (2001), review	39 studies, community, clinic and hospital settings, adults and older people (n = 20 218)	11% (major diagnostic interview) 31% (rating scales)
Multiple sclerosis		
Chwastiak et al. (2002)	Community sample (n = 739)	29%

TABLE 6.1 (CONTINUED)

*By diagnostic interview or validated scale.
†Type 1 and type 2.
CHD, coronary heart disease; COPD, chronic obstructive pulmonary disease.

Anderson RJ, Freedland KE, Clouse RE, Lustman PJ. The prevalence of comorbid depression in adults with diabetes: a meta-analysis. *Diabetes Care* 2001;24:1069–78.

Chwastiak L, Ehde DM, Gibbons LE et al. Depressive symptoms and severity of illness in multiple sclerosis: epidemiologic study of a large community sample. *Am J Psychiatry* 2002;159:1862–8.

Lett HS, Blumenthal JA, Babyak MA et al. Depression as a risk factor for coronary artery disease: evidence, mechanisms, and treatment. *Psychosom Med* 2004;66:305–15.

Robinson RG. Poststroke depression: prevalence, diagnosis, treatment, and disease progression. *Biol Psychiatry* 2003;54:376–87.

Rudisch B, Nemeroff CB. Epidemiology of comorbid coronary artery disease and depression. *Biol Psychiatry* 2003;54:227–40.

van Ede L, Yzermans CJ, Brouwer HJ. Prevalence of depression in patients with chronic obstructive pulmonary disease: a systematic review. *Thorax* 1999;54:688–92.

Wagena EJ, van Amelsvoort LG, Kant I, Wouters EF. Chronic bronchitis, cigarette smoking, and the subsequent onset of depression and anxiety: results from a prospective population-based cohort study. *Psychosom Med* 2005;67:656–60.

Weintraub D, Oehlberg KA, Katz IR, Stern MB. Test characteristics of the 15-item geriatric depression scale and Hamilton depression rating scale in Parkinson disease. *Am J Geriatr Psychiatry* 2006;14:169–75.

Adapted from Tylee A, Haddad M. Managing complex problems: treatment for common mental disorders in the UK. *Epidemiol Psichiatr Soc* 2007;16:302–8.

or, vice versa, medical illness may relate to adverse effects of depression treatment.

It is likely that the association involves a number of mechanisms that may act and interact simultaneously, and many of the linkages appear to be bi-directional. For example, a meta-analysis of relevant study findings has shown the link between depression and obesity to be reciprocal: obesity was found to increase the risk of depression, but also depression is predictive of developing obesity.

Depression as a predictor of physical illness

Depression may increase the likelihood of developing certain medical conditions; evidence from longitudinal studies involving occupational and geographic cohorts shows most clearly that a history of depression is linked to developing cardiovascular disease and to the onset of diabetes. Cohort studies conducted in the USA and Japan also show that depression is an independent risk factor for stroke. There is weaker evidence that links depression to the incidence of cancer and hypertension.

There seem to be two main mechanisms involved in linking depression to later medical illness (and to worsened outcomes from these illnesses such as increased mortality). These are behavioral and physiological, though their effects are likely to be interlinked.

Studies have shown that people with minor and major depression are less likely to engage in leisure-time physical activity or to adhere to medical treatments (for example, eye examinations or flu injections in an adult diabetic population), and are more likely to be current cigarette smokers. Physical inactivity, poor diet, reduced adherence to medication regimens, and smoking may be influenced by features of depression such as reduced interest and pleasure, lack of energy and diminished motivation; and these are clear risks for the development and exacerbation of medical illness. Physical inactivity appears to be a very important factor linking heart disease and depression, with recent studies identifying that a substantial proportion of the association between depressive symptoms and cardiovascular events is accounted for by lack of exercise.

Depression has particular effects on physiological processes that can underlie the relationship with medical illnesses. These include changes in the hypothalamic–pituitary–adrenal axis function – most notably in cortisol secretion, which affects immune system function and inflammatory responses. Various aspects of inflammatory function, including altered cytokines, appear to lead to atherosclerosis. Additionally, abnormalities in neurotransmitter metabolism have been linked to changes in platelet aggregation, and associated effects on autonomic nervous system function are linked to decreased heart rate variability, all of which predispose patients to cardiac events. The development of diabetes following depression, and the relationship between depression and glycemic control wherein it is associated with persistently higher HbA_{1c} levels appears to be linked to changed plasma glucocorticoid levels decreasing insulin sensitivity.

Physical illness predicting depression

The most intuitively plausible link between physical illness and depression is that the stresses, role limitations and pain related to a medical condition may cause depression. However, clarifying this relationship is complicated by the fact that depression onset, which is typically in early adulthood, usually occurs many years before the development of chronic medical conditions, which are generally rare before middle age. But there have been studies that follow participants without depression and examine the risk of depression incidence in relation to physical illnesses. Reviews of relevant studies have found an elevated risk of depression among people who have been diagnosed with asthma, chronic obstructive pulmonary disease (COPD), cancer, diabetes, arthritis and heart disease; a systematic review of 20 prospective studies indicates that the increased risk is related to the disabling impacts of these diseases and their effects on sleep. The effects of disability as a risk factor for depression are most commonly identified in older people, but appear to operate across the age range. Although a range of factors are likely to be involved, persistent pain has been found to be an important predictor of depression.

For some neurological and endocrine conditions, it appears that particular physiological processes may operate to elevate depression risk – for example, through cerebrovascular changes, which may be implicated in heart disease, diabetes and stroke, or degenerative changes in the brain as occur in Alzheimer's disease and Parkinson's disease.

Additional linkages: predisposing factors and treatment side effects

Shared genetic factors that increase the risk for both depression and particular physical conditions such as diabetes or heart disease may play a part in the relationship between medical conditions and depression. A number of research programs are exploring this topic, and emerging evidence indicates that genetically influenced pathways linking these conditions are highly likely, and that – as for many other health problems – there is an interaction between multiple genetic factors and environmental factors. There is clear evidence that social and economic adversity and traumatic early childhood experiences such as physical, psychological or sexual abuse and emotional neglect are linked to a heightened risk of both medical illness and depression. Patterns of coping and ways of responding to stressors that develop in the first years of life and are powerfully influenced by early environment appear to act as further predisposing and perpetuating factors for these health problems.

Additionally, depressive disorders can occur primarily as a side effect of the treatment of a physical disorder. Commonly prescribed medications such as analgesics, antihypertensive drugs, steroids, antiparkinsonian agents and interferon treatment for hepatitis C may have this potential adverse effect. On the other hand, antidepressant medications are associated with weight gain and metabolic abnormalities, including insulin resistance and elevated serum lipid concentrations in vulnerable patients, and these drugs have also been linked to hypertension and adverse bone mineral density changes.

Understanding the mechanisms that link depression and physical illness is clearly important for designing the types of intervention that will be most effective for prevention and treatment. Further knowledge of these linkages may lead to more accurate screening tests (possibly based on biomarkers of risk), better targeted health education and promotion, more effective programs to assist changes in behavior, and more appropriate treatment decisions.

Chronic diseases

Although many medical illnesses are associated with increased depression prevalence, there is a particularly strong association with chronic diseases. This is a group of non-communicable diseases, including type 2 diabetes, coronary heart disease, hypertension, stroke, COPD and end-stage renal disease. They have multiple and often shared causal risk factors, typically there is a long interval between risk exposure and symptom development, and there is characteristically a sustained illness period that ultimately results in disability. For all these conditions there is a two- to threefold increased prevalence of depression compared with the unaffected population.

There are geographic variations in the rates of these conditions, and their prevalence is influenced by socioeconomic factors, sex and ethnicity. However, age appears to be the most important factor affecting the prevalence of long-term conditions, and the demographic changes in the world population are leading to a sustained increase in these conditions and the burden of disease attributable to them. Long-term conditions are becoming increasingly common in all the world regions, primarily because of changes in global demographics. Recent WHO data reveal that 60% of all deaths worldwide and 43% of the global burden of disease are attributable to chronic diseases, and projections indicate that over the next decade chronic diseases are expected to account for nearly three-quarters (73%) of all deaths and 60% of the global burden of disease.

People with long-term conditions use much more healthcare than those without such conditions, with around a doubling for primary care consultations and specialist appointments; the highest increases are for those elements of healthcare that are the most costly (i.e. inpatient bed days). Many of those people with a chronic medical problem report having two or more conditions: this is the case for around 50% of people with chronic illness. This co-occurrence of multiple chronic diseases is termed multimorbidity, and surveys conducted in the USA, Canada, Australia and European countries identify that its likelihood increases with age, and that it is related to reduced function and poorer quality of life.

Approaches to assessment and management

The global changes in the distribution and prevalence of chronic illnesses will have important effects on the level and focus required of our health policies and services. Because of the strong relationship between these conditions and depression, there are particular challenges in developing the necessary resources, knowledge and skills to meet the needs of people with this combination of problems. There is a clear need for better integration of mental health assessment and practice across the healthcare system.

Healthcare professionals in primary and secondary medical care encounter a large (and increasing) number of people whose physical illnesses are complicated by mental health problems, and skills and confidence in assessing and monitoring symptoms and negotiating appropriate care are vital. Conversely, mental health professionals' skills in identifying and promoting evidence-based management for physical health problems is increasingly recognized as an essential part of their role, as is the need for these staff to provide relevant support and supervision for their primary care colleagues in the management of comorbidity.

Increased awareness of the mental health needs of patients irrespective of disease categories is necessary in the training of personnel and the planning of services, so that mental health problems such as depression are appropriately recognized and managed. Being able to identify depression in combination with long-term medical illnesses is an essential first step to ongoing monitoring and agreeing approaches to problem management, but this is complicated by a number of factors. The patient's expectations and attitudes influence the help-seeking process, and stigma and uncertainty about psychological problems may lead to medical illness features being expressed more freely than emotional difficulties. The clinician may similarly be more comfortable with eliciting physical rather than psychological problems. Limited consultation duration and the means of service payment or reimbursement may additionally steer the encounter towards the review and management of medical conditions. There are also difficulties related to interpreting some of the presenting symptoms, because the physical or somatic features of depression, such as fatigue and psychomotor retardation, disturbed appetite and weight loss, and poor sleep, may result from the medical condition or its treatment, and the possibility of depression as a reason for the symptoms may not be considered. Possible confusion arising from multiple causes of symptoms has led some workers to advocate discounting physical symptoms when assessing comorbid depression. However, the evidence from investigations of the validity of diagnostic practice indicates that modifications to depression criteria are not an appropriate response to these problems. Somatic symptoms retain their importance in assessing depression in people with physical disease, and a full assessment of all clinical features, together with relevant history and social factors, and including the person's own understanding of his or her problems, is always required.

Identification. There are a number of depression case identification (or screening) tools available to assist practice in this area. As part of the development of recent National Institute for Health and Clinical Excellence (NICE) guidance (for England, Wales and Northern Ireland), a systematic review has been undertaken of the adequacy of depression case identification instruments within this population. Evidence indicates that for people in primary care or general hospital settings, those with chronic physical health problems, including older people, the most commonly used measures – such as the Hospital Anxiety and Depression Scale, the Geriatric Depression Scale, the Beck Depression Inventory, the Centre for Epidemiological Studies Depression Scale and the Patient Health Questionnaire (PHQ-9) – all perform adequately. A simply administered two-question screen appears to have excellent sensitivity, and is an appropriate tool for initial assessment and routine monitoring (see Table 4.2, page 59). Recognition of depression is covered in more detail in Chapter 4.

Management. There are well-founded concerns that standard guidance for the management of depression is inappropriate for people who experience depression together with medical conditions, because of uncertainty about the effectiveness of routine treatments for these people, and the risks of side effects and drug interactions related to these conditions and their treatments. Although the presence of comorbid medical illness complicates treatment decisions, there is a strong evidence base to guide practice, with antidepressant and psychological treatments shown to be effective for depression and improving quality of life across many disorders – from diabetes and heart disease to cancer and COPD. Recent NICE guidance notes that selective serotonin reuptake inhibitors are an appropriate first-line drug treatment. Sertraline and citalopram are the probable drugs of first choice on the basis of lower interaction potential and safety in relation to cardiac events.

As for depression in the absence of physical illness, a range of psychosocial interventions have been found to be effective. Lower-intensity interventions such as guided self-help, relaxation training and exercise are beneficial in milder forms of depression, while individual and group cognitive and behavioral therapies appear to be an appropriate option for treating more severe forms of depression combined with medical illness. Chapter 5 explores treatment options in greater detail.

Key points – combined with physical health problems

- Depression is two to three times more common among people experiencing medical conditions, as physical illness increases the risks for depression and, vice versa, depression makes physical illness more likely.
- When depression and physical illnesses are combined the course and outcome of both conditions are worsened, with increased disability, higher medical costs and greater likelihood of adverse outcomes (including death).
- People with depression are less likely to adhere to treatments for medical conditions or to adopt healthy behaviors and self-management for these health problems.
- Recognizing depression in people with physical health problems can be challenging, but being alert to the increased risk and using validated case-finding measures assists this process.
- There is a good evidence base for managing depression combined with medical conditions: selective serotonin reuptake inhibitors (SSRIs) are an appropriate first-line drug treatment and psychological therapies are effective.

Key references

See also Table 6.1

Das-Munshi J, Stewart R, Ismail K et al. Diabetes, common mental disorders, and disability: findings from the UK National Psychiatric Morbidity Survey. *Psychosom Med* 2007;69:543–50.

Haddad M. Caring for patients with long-term conditions and depression. *Nurs Stand* 2010;24:40–9; quiz 50.

Moussavi S, Chatterji S, Verdes E et al. Depression, chronic diseases, and decrements in health: results from the World Health Surveys. *Lancet* 2007;370:851–8.

National Institute for Health and Clinical Excellence. *Depression in Adults with a Chronic Physical Health Problem: Treatment and Management (Clinical Guideline 91).* London: National Institute for Health and Clinical Excellence, 2009.

Prince M, Patel V, Saxena S et al. No health without mental health. *Lancet* 2007;370:859–77.

7 / Self-harm and suicide

I don't like standing near the edge of a platform when an express train is passing through. I like to stand right back and if possible get a pillar between me and the train. I don't like to stand by the side of a ship and look down into the water. A second's action would end everything. A few drops of desperation

Winston Churchill

Suicide is a major public health problem. It accounts for nearly one million deaths in the world, and in the US twice as many people die by suicide as by homicide. International data reveal that currently around four times as many people die from suicide as from war or civil conflicts (World Health Report, 2004). In the last 45 years suicide rates have increased by 60% worldwide, and it is now one of the three leading causes of death among 15–44 year-olds. Deaths from suicide are projected by the WHO to increase to over 1.5 million by 2020.

There are wide variations in the suicide rates for different countries and regions, with highest rates in the Baltic States and sub-Saharan Africa, and lowest in Latin America. Suicide is the eleventh leading cause of death in the USA, accounting for 33 300 deaths in 2006, with an overall rate of 10.9 suicide deaths per 100 000 people; this compares with a rate (in 2006) of 30.1 per 100 000 in the Russian Federation (42 855 deaths).

Suicide rates are much higher among men than women in practically all regions of the world. Until recently, suicide was most common among older men but changes in suicide rates have led to young men becoming the group at highest risk, with suicides in this group predominating in absolute and relative terms in a third of all countries.

Many more people make suicide attempts or self-harming acts than kill themselves: self-harm is estimated to be 20 times more common than suicide, and a history of self-harm is an important risk factor for completed suicide. The reasons for suicide are complex and vary with age, sex, culture and ethnicity. Many of these factors are best understood in the context of each person's individual life and life circumstances.

Definitions

A number of terms are used in the literature to define suicide acts, with a lack of consistency creating some problems in collating and comparing relevant data from different countries.

- Suicide: the act of deliberately killing oneself; it is a fatal suicidal act.
- Self-harm: a range of terms are widely used, including parasuicide, attempted suicide, non-fatal suicidal acts, self-harm, deliberate self-harm or self-injury.

Aside from the potential for confusion resulting from the range of terms that apply to self-harming activity, there is a problem in the implied intention, with those terms incorporating suicide linking the action to a purpose. The broader term 'self-harm' avoids any such assumption, and is defined as an act with a non-fatal outcome in which an individual deliberately tries to harm themselves.

Recent guidance for the National Health Service in England, Wales and Northern Ireland (NICE 2004) notes that self-harm is "An expression of personal distress usually made in private by an individual who hurts him/herself. The nature and meaning of self-harm may vary greatly from person to person. The reasons a person harms him/herself may be different on each occasion and should not be presumed to be the same."

Self-harm most commonly involves harm by cutting or by ingesting a substance in excess of the generally recognized therapeutic dose (self-poisoning).

Epidemiology of suicide

Global rate increases. Although there has been a marked rise in the global rate of suicide since 1950, the extent of this must be addressed with some caution as the data from which the baseline rate was derived were very limited: 11 countries provided data for the WHO suicide mortality databank in 1950, but this had increased to more than 70 countries by the 1980s, and the rates in the more recently included countries are likely to be higher than those in the initial group. Additionally, changes in the former Soviet Union have been associated with former USSR states reporting high suicide rates.

Age trends. Global data show a clear picture of the rising prevalence of completed suicide with age. Worldwide, older people have the highest rate of completed suicide rate of any age group, with the pooled international rate increasing gradually from 1.2 (per 100 000 males) in the 5–14 year-old age group to 55.7 in the over-75 years group (Figure 7.1). For women, the rate increases less steeply to 18.8 per 100 000 females.

Despite this marked difference in rates of suicide, examination of the number of people dying by suicide shows that more young people are dying than old: more than 55% of global suicides occur in people younger than 45 years.

Over the last few decades, there has been a rising trend of youth suicide. In 21 of the 30 countries in the WHO European region, suicide rates in young men aged 15–19 rose between 1979 and 1996;

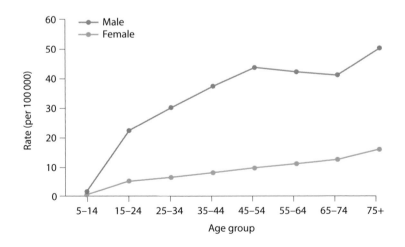

Figure 7.1 Distribution of suicide rates, by sex, in 2000: WHO pooled data. From WHO, 2002.

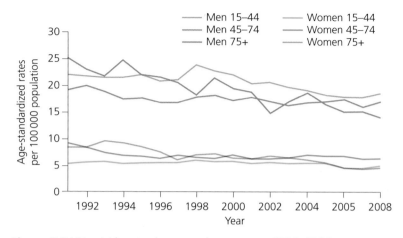

Figure 7.2 UK suicide rates by sex and age group, 1991–2008.
Source: Office for National Statistics, www.statistics.gov.uk/cci/nugget.
asp?id=1092, last accessed 15 July 2011. Crown Copyright material is
reproduced with the permission of the Office of Public Sector Information
(OPSI).

further examination of age-specific rates shows that suicide rates
among young males (under 45 years) have risen whilst rates among
the older men (55 and over) have declined. Against a background
of suicide rates that have been stable or falling in many industrialized
countries, this rise in suicide for young males appears particularly
marked.

Similar trends are apparent in the suicide data from the UK,
Australia and the USA, where the rates of suicide among young men
increased from around 1970 until the early or mid-1990s, but have
subsequently declined. In England and Wales, rates of suicide in men
under 45 years doubled in the years to 1998 when they reached the
highest level since the 1920s. The recent trends for UK suicide rates
are shown in Figure 7.2.

The relative rates of suicides within specific age groups differs
markedly in particular countries and regions: in Australia, the UK and
the USA, the rate in the 15–19 years age group is close to the mean
rate for the country, while in Russia the rate among this age group is
more than three times higher than the mean rate. In Sri Lanka, the

suicide rate in the 15–19 years age group is more than six times the mean rate for this country (and around four to six times the rate in the UK, USA and Australia).

Sex. In almost all world regions and across all age groups, suicide is three to four times higher in men than in women. This characteristic sex difference is markedly reduced in Asian countries such as India and Hong Kong, where a ratio of less than two is observed. In rural China, there is an increased rate of suicide among women compared to men, and this is strongest in young women aged 20–34 years. Several other non-European countries – Sri Lanka, El Salvador, Cuba and Ecuador – have suicide rates for young women aged 15–19 years that exceed those of young men in the same age group.

Geographic variations. There are large-scale variations in suicide prevalence between nations and cultures, with the highest rates currently evident in the countries of the Russian Federation and Eastern Europe, and the lowest in the Eastern Mediterranean region and Latin America. Additionally, high rates are evident in several island countries: Sri Lanka, Japan, Cuba and Mauritius. Figure 7.3 shows the most recent global suicide rates available at the time of press.

The reasons for these geographic differences in suicide rates relate to many variables, including the following.

Access to lethal agents that can be means of suicide appears an important factor, with observational evidence from the UK showing a marked reduction in suicide rates associated with change of domestic gas supply from toxic town gas to non-toxic natural gas. Similarly, the high suicide rates evident in rural China and other Asian regions may be related to the ready availability of highly toxic pesticides.

Upheavals in political and economic systems may result in diminished social integration, instability and uncertainty about the future. The stark increases in suicide rates observed in Russia and the former Soviet republics since the 1990s provide an indication of the relationship between economic circumstances, social cohesion and suicide, which was first considered by Durkheim more than a century ago.

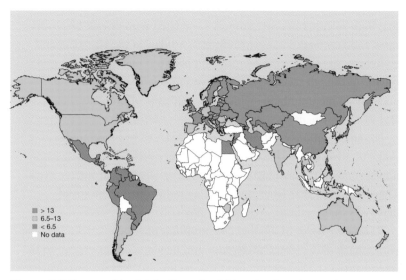

Figure 7.3 Geographic distribution of suicide rates (most recent year available as of 2009). Reproduced with permission from WHO (www.who. int/mental_health/prevention/suicide/suicideprevent/en, last accessed 15 July 2011).

Religious beliefs or the prevailing religious denomination in a culture may act to reduce suicide acts, indeed some religions expressively forbid suicide. Current data indicate that suicide rates are highest in atheist nations (26 per 100 000) such as China, and lowest in Islamic countries (near zero). Hindu and Christian countries have rates around the median (11 per 100 000), and in Buddhist countries such as Japan the rates are high (18 per 100 000).

Suicide acts motivated by the desire to kill others have occurred in several wars and have become more widespread in the conflicts in Sri Lanka, Iraq, Palestine and Afghanistan. In the Second World War such acts were prominent as a tactic of the Japanese forces, being linked to both Samurai tradition and imperial decree; contemporary suicide bombings as a response to foreign occupation are strongly associated with Islamic ideology where they are seen as an act of martyrdom.

Unemployment, poverty, and residential instability are associated with suicide in observational analyses within and between nations. Recent analysis of data from 25 European Union countries indicates that high suicide rates are strongly correlated with at-risk-of-poverty rates and low healthcare expenditures. Studies in the UK, USA and elsewhere reveal a strong relationship between unemployment and suicide (although some of this association is confounded by the presence of mental illness, which is a predictor of both suicide and unemployment).

Income inequality within nations appears to be associated with a range of adverse health and social outcomes such as homicide rates, imprisonment, teenage births, obesity, drug misuse and suicide rates. These effects appear to be mediated by reductions in the social networks that facilitate civic engagement.

Rates and styles of alcohol consumption may be related to suicide, with a nation's beverage preference and drinking culture noted to be significant in studies examining these factors in Norway, Sweden, France, Denmark and Portugal. Heavy drinking and binge drinking – particularly when involving spirits – appear to be associated with raised suicide rates.

Depression and suicide

The data on the association between suicide, mental disorder and service use are derived from studies almost entirely conducted in Europe and the USA. Hence, caution is required if extrapolating to other regions. Reviews of these findings show that 90% of suicide completers have a diagnosable mental disorder, though fewer have had contact with mental health services in the year before suicide, around 30%. Depression seems to be the most important disease risk factor for suicidal ideation and behavior among all age groups, and is present in around 60% of completed cases. Other mental disorders that are particularly strongly associated with suicide are: bipolar affective disorder, schizophrenia, alcohol dependence and addiction to other substances.

Although the rate of suicide in people with depression in the USA and UK is often quoted as 15%, this figure is based on a selective sample of patients with severe depression. The lifetime risk for suicide among people treated as inpatients for depression is around 4%, while that for those treated as outpatients is 2%. Depression together with alcoholism is the combination most frequently found in population studies that have recorded multiple diagnoses.

Hopelessness is strongly linked to the presence of suicidal ideation. Additionally, family conflict, serious physical illness and loneliness are all associated with completed suicide.

Risk factors for suicide

There is general agreement between research evidence and clinical experience that the two key risk factors for suicide are:

- the presence of one or more diagnosable mental disorder, particularly depression, occurring alone or comorbid with a substance misuse disorders
- a prior suicide attempt.

More general factors associated with suicide include:

- a family history of mental disorder
- a family history of suicide, or other exposure to suicidal behavior involving family or peers or in media reports or fictional representations
- family violence, including physical or sexual abuse
- impulsiveness – characterized as involving impetuous actions, reduced attention and a lack of future planning
- being in custody or the care system
- male sex
- divorce or separation
- unemployment
- poor physical health.

Suicide in prisoners. In the UK and USA, the age-standardized rates of suicide among people in prison are, respectively, five and eight times higher than those for the general population. A recent systematic review of risk factors, based on nearly 5000 prison suicides in prisons in 12 countries, has identified that risk is strongly associated with:

- recent suicidal ideation
- being accommodated in a single cell
- a history of attempted suicide

- evidence of a mental disorder or being prescribed psychotropic medication
- detainee or remand status
- a history of alcohol misuse problems.

In common with the general population, male sex conferred higher risk, while in contrast being married was inversely associated with suicide for prisoners.

These risk factors provide crucial information to inform prison suicide prevention strategies, by enhancing the ability of staff to identify predictors. Importantly, several of the factors are potentially modifiable and can inform intervention approaches for these vulnerable individuals.

Self-harm

People who die by suicide represent only a fraction of the number who harm themselves in response to life problems or contemplate suicide. Acts of self-harm are relatively common, particularly among young people. They are usually related to life problems and intended to cause harm (but not serious or permanent) rather than endanger life. This notwithstanding, self-harm acts are a strong predictor of future suicidal behavior, and require careful and sensitive assessment and management.

Epidemiology. Self-harm is far more common among adolescents than any other age group. A recent large-scale survey of 15 and 16 year olds in English schools using anonymous self-report questionnaires indicated that nearly 9% had self-harmed in the past year, and that 13% had a lifetime history of self-harm. This behavior is more common in adolescent girls who were found to be nearly four times more likely than boys to self-harm.

A recent systematic review of self-harm behavior in adolescence involving data from over 500000 adolescents indicated nearly 10% had harmed themselves, while nearly 30% of adolescents said they had thought about suicide at some point.

The most recent Adult Psychiatric Morbidity Survey in England (2007) found that among this whole population, between 5% and 6%

reported ever engaging in self-harm, and 17% of people reported that they had thought about committing suicide at some point in their life.

A higher frequency of self-harm in adolescence is correlated with the consumption of cigarettes or alcohol and the number of times drunk (particularly in females), and all categories of drug misuse. It is also associated with being bullied and with physical and sexual abuse. Many young people report repeated self-harm, and such repetition has been found most commonly in the presence of mental health problems or significant psychosocial disadvantages.

A history of self-harm is the strongest predictor of future suicide, increasing the risk by 50–100-fold compared with people who have not self-harmed. A systematic review found that 16% of patients who attended an emergency department because of self-harm repeated this behavior, and 1.8% died by suicide.

Evidence from the UK and Sweden shows that people who use more dangerous methods to harm themselves (such as hanging, using firearms or gas, jumping from heights or using more lethal poisons) are at higher risk of subsequent suicide.

Management of self-harm. It is crucial to ensure that front-line services are equipped to address the needs of people who self-harm in an effective manner. Sensitive and comprehensive risk assessment is of central importance. The response of some health professionals to people who self-harm has been found to be intolerant and critical, and changing the awareness and attitudes of staff through training is part of professional and service development in many settings. It is vital that professionals in emergency departments, primary care, schools, prisons and hospital wards are aware of best practice guidance and show willingness to provide help at the point at which people request it.

It may be necessary to raise awareness among professionals (e.g. working in health, schools and prisons) about people who may find it difficult to seek help, such as older men, people from ethnic minority communities and gay men, and to test opportunistic and organized approaches to increase identification of these at-risk groups.

TABLE 7.1

Risk assessment following self-harm

- Review the attempt – was there suicide ideation; was the intention to die; were lethal means used?
- Review mental state – assess for depression and other mental disorder, and for substance misuse.
- Are there current suicidal ideas; is there intention and a plan?
- Review past history – have there been previous suicidal behaviors; is there a family history of mental disorder, suicide or self-harm?
- Review family and relationship factors – are there relationship problems; loss or bereavement; family discord; is there abuse (emotional/sexual/physical); are there sexual identity difficulties?
- Review social and environmental factors: employment/attending education; difficulties at work/school – isolation, bullying, disaffection?
- Review support networks and any past treatment – consider engagement and motivation to change, ability to collaborate in short- and medium-term plans and take responsibility for safety?

Table 7.1 shows the main elements of risk assessment procedure for individuals who present following self-harm.

Suicide prevention programs

A strategy for suicide prevention requires increased awareness about suicidal behaviors and approaches to their prevention. This is particularly important within primary care because many people seek medical care in the month before their suicide, providing a clear window of opportunity for intervention. Improved knowledge and awareness is also necessary across a range of sectors – such as schools and colleges, prisons, counseling centers and alcohol and substance misuse support services, and within the media. Prevention strategies should also incorporate efforts to reduce the availability of and access to means of suicide (e.g. toxic substances, such as medicines or pesticides).

The assessment and monitoring of risk of suicide is an important aspect of depression care, and must be explicitly evaluated for all patients who appear depressed. The skills to engage and sensitively assess and monitor this risk are necessary for all professionals who work with people who may be depressed, particularly because there is a potential for increased risk in the early stages of treatment. Interventions aimed at primary care professionals and other 'frontline' health staff designed to increase identification of people at risk of suicide have been developed in a number of countries, and there is evidence that training practitioners can improve the identification of those patients at risk. A systematic review recently found that physician education in depression recognition and management and restricting access to lethal methods reduces suicide rates.

Approaches to improve awareness of populations at risk (such as prisoners, older people, young people in care), and to provide support and management appropriate to their particular needs must be part of national and local suicide prevention plans.

Key points – self-harm and suicide

- Suicide is strongly associated with depression, but despite depression being more common among adult women, men are around three to four times more likely than women to kill themselves in most countries of the world.
- Self-harm is most common in adolescent girls and young women and usually does not involve an intention to endanger life; nonetheless a history of self-harm is an important predictor of future suicide, increasing the risk by 50–100-fold compared with people who have not self-harmed.
- In addition to previous self-harm, risk factors for suicide include depression, substance misuse, a family history of suicide, male sex, being separated or divorced, and being in custody.
- Assessment practice following self-harm needs to be sensitive and skilled, focusing on the presence of risk factors for suicide and basing care plans on clearly defined risks and the capacity of the individual and their support network to manage problems and take responsibility for safety.

Key references

Bernal M, Haro JM, Bernert S et al. Risk factors for suicidality in Europe: results from the ESEMED study. *J Affect Disord* 2007;101: 27–34.

Biddle L, Brock A, Brookes ST, Gunnell D. Suicide rates in young men in England and Wales in the 21st century: time trend study. *BMJ* 2008;336:539–42.

Blair-West GW, Mellsop GW, Eyeson-Annan ML. Down-rating lifetime suicide risk in major depression. *Acta Psychiatr Scand* 1997;95:259–63.

De Leo D, Heller TS. Who are the kids who self-harm? An Australian self-report school survey. *Med J Aust* 2004;181:140–4.

Dumesnil H, Verger P. Public awareness campaigns about depression and suicide: a review. *Psychiatr Serv* 2009;60:1203–13.

Evans E, Hawton K, Rodham K, Deeks J. The prevalence of suicidal phenomena in adolescents: a systematic review of population-based studies. *Suicide Life Threat Behav* 2005;35:239–50.

Fazel S, Cartwright J, Norman-Nott A, Hawton K. Suicide in prisoners: a systematic review of risk factors. *J Clin Psychiatry* 2008;69:1721–31.

Gask L, Dixon C, Morriss R, Appleby L, Green G. Evaluating STORM skills training for managing people at risk of suicide. *J Adv Nurs* 2006;54:739–50.

Gould MS, Greenberg T, Velting DM, Shaffer D. Youth suicide risk and preventive interventions: a review of the past 10 years. *J Am Acad Child Adolesc Psychiatry* 2003;42:386–405.

Hawton K. Completed suicide after attempted suicide. *BMJ* 2010; 341:c3064.

National Institute for Health and Clinical Excellence. *Self-harm: The Short-term Physical and Psychological Management and Secondary Prevention of Self-Harm in Primary and Secondary Care (Clinical Guideline 16).* London: National Institute for Health and Clinical Excellence, 2004.

Paton J, Jenkins R, Scott J. Collective approaches for the control of depression in England. *Soc Psychiatry Psychiatr Epidemiol* 2001;36:423–8.

World Health Organization. *Suicide Prevention (SUPRE).* Geneva: WHO, 2002. Available from www. who.int/mental_health/prevention/ suicide/suicideprevent/en/, last accessed 15 July 2011.

Useful resources

UK
Association for Postnatal
Depression
http://apni.org

**Aware – helping to defeat
depression**
Information and support for
people with depression in Ireland
and Northern Ireland
www.aware.ie

Depression Alliance
Information, resources, links, and
news about local events, including
self-help groups
www.depressionalliance.org

Depression UK
UK support group for people
suffering from depression
info@depressionuk.org
www.depressionuk.org

Healthtalkonline
www.healthtalkonline.org/mental_
health

Living Life to the Full
Free access to online mental health
life skills course based on CBT
www.llttf.com

**MDF The BiPolar Organisation/
The BiPolar Organisation Cymru**
A user-led charity for people with
bipolar disorder
mdf@mdf.org.uk and
info@mdfwales.org.uk
www.mdf.org.uk and
www.mdfwales.org.uk

Mental Health Foundation
Information on problems,
treatments and strategies, news
and events
www.mentalhealth.org.uk

**MIND (National Association for
Mental Health)**
Information and self-help on
depression, related issues for all
mental health problems
www.mind.org.uk

Relate
The UK's largest relationship
counseling organization
enquiries@relate.org.uk
www.relate.org.uk

Royal College of Psychiatrists

Readable and well-researched information for the public – wide range of leaflets and other resources.
www.rcpsych.ac.uk/
mentalhealthinfoforall/problems/
depression.aspx

Samaritans

National organization offering support to people in distress who feel suicidal or despairing
Helpline: 08457 90 90 90
jo@samaritans.org
www.samaritans.org

SaneLine

A national out-of-hours telephone helpline offering emotional support and information. Open from 6 PM to 11 PM every day
Tel: 0845 767 8000
www.sane.org.uk

Young Minds

UK charity concerned with improving children and young peoples' mental health (under 25s). Web pages for young people at www.youngminds.org.uk/young-people
www.youngminds.org.uk

USA

Mental Health America

Provider of support, public education and advocacy
www.nmha.org

National Alliance on Mental Illness

Offering support, education, advocacy and research
www.nami.org

National Institute of Mental Health

Depression information, publications, research and links
www.nimh.nih.gov/health/topics/
depression/index.shtml

Australia

beyondblue (the national depression initiative)

www.beyondblue.org.au

Blackdog Institute

A not-for-profit educational, research, clinical and community-oriented facility offering specialist expertise in depression and bipolar disorder
www.blackdoginstitute.org.au

DepressioNet
Self-help website
http://depressioNet.org.au

Moodgym
Developed in Australia, Moodgym
is a free interactive program for
anxiety and depression based on
CBT and IPT
http://moodgym.anu.edu.au

National Prescribing Service
http://www.nps.org.au

Reach Out
Information and tools for young
people
http://au.reachout.com

Index